D1362590

528 175 19 9

MICHELLE ELMAN is a five-board accredited body confidence coach and body positive activist. She has appeared on Sky News, Channel 4 News, BBC Radio London, BBC Radio 5 Live, LBC, and has been featured in over three hundred press articles worldwide. Her TedX talk titled 'Have You Hated Your Body Enough Today?' has been viewed over 40,000 times.

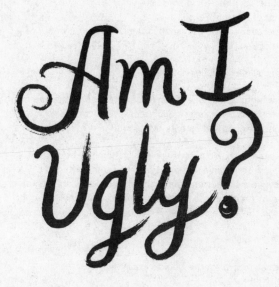

# Am I Ugly?

MICHELLE ELMAN

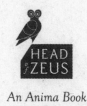

HEAD
of
ZEUS

*An Anima Book*

First published in the UK in 2018 by Anima,
an imprint of Head of Zeus Ltd
This paperback edition published in the UK in 2019
by Head of Zeus Ltd

9 7 5 3 1 2 4 6 8

A catalogue record for this book is available from
the British Library.

ISBN (PB): 9781788541855
ISBN (E): 9781788541831

Typeset by Adrian McLaughlin

Printed and bound in Great Britain by
CPI Group (UK) Ltd, Croydon CR0 4YY

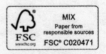

Head of Zeus Ltd
First Floor East
5–8 Hardwick Street
London EC1R 4RG

WWW.HEADOFZEUS.COM

*For every child that is lying in a hospital bed wondering what they did to deserve this – you aren't alone.*

# CONTENTS

# AUTHOR'S NOTE

Some of the names of both people and places in this book have been changed in order to protect the dignity and privacy of the innocent – and particularly, the not-so innocent. Identifying details about individuals and locations have also been changed, but the stories that are told within this book are all factual and accurate to my recollection.

The events that occur are exactly how I remember them happening at the time; however, as with any story, my experience will be biased by my own perceptions. This is my most authentic truth and I take solace in knowing that I would be the villain in someone else's story but for now, this is mine.

# SECTION ONE

# 1

## Am I being a drama queen?

My school uniform – a kilt and pinstriped shirt – was clinging to the carpet. The lavender tie around my neck was tangled and trapped under my elbow, restraining me even further. I felt a prickling sensation on my face where it had hit the floor – and my head was throbbing. It took a while for the sounds of the room to return. I heard the girls screaming, and then I heard them being silenced.

Footsteps approached slowly.

It was Mrs Wright, my teacher.

'Stand up.'

I had fainted at school, the second time in the week. It was my first year at boarding school in England. I was just eleven, a small and skinny girl with a tight ponytail and bright pink and purple glasses. There had been the usual stresses of adjustment to a new school and being away from home for the first time, and these had been compounded by migraines. Terrible migraines. The week before, as term exams approached, the pain had been so excruciating that I'd had difficulty standing. In the nurse's office I was given a painkiller and a cool cloth for my head and sent on my way, back to class. Later, when I became dizzy and fainted, I was taken to the medical centre for further examination. The diagnosis: I was coming down with the flu.

When the flu didn't come, I returned to class and fainted again. I was taken to see another doctor, who diagnosed my problem as emotional. Stress was the culprit. The mega-hothouse climate of St Keyes, where girls from all over the world came to a remote and boggy corner of the British Isles to receive a traditional education and compete with each other on a microscopic level in every aspect of their lives – academically, socially, musically, right down to who had the best handwriting – was to blame. The school motto: Trust, Encouragement and Mutual Respect, which was drilled into us constantly, to the point of misery, had done little to mitigate the pressure.

The doctor had declared that I was stressed from the workload and exams and told me to take it easy, try to relax, and rest. I did as I was told – or as much as a St Keyes girl knew how to rest. While I spent the entire weekend in bed, my friends took turns sitting beside me and helping me review my course material and study. Exams, just a little more than a week away, were considered the benchmark of the entire year; so while I could rest my body physically, my brain couldn't take the same kind of break. With this in mind, I began attending class again.

That morning, a Saturday, I was preparing for chapel when I began to feel weak again. I visited the nurse who gave me a painkiller, slapped a futile 'cooling strip' across my forehead and told me that I needed to return to class. But the throbbing in my head was excruciating. I walked to class crying.

What I haven't yet explained is that having a so-called 'headache' wasn't new to me. It's not that I was used to them – you never get used to that kind of knives-in-the-brain pain – but I'd been having them ever since I could remember. I have a condition called hydrocephalus, which is an excess of cerebrospinal fluid. This condition had led to a series of surgeries when I was younger, the last being when I was seven, in order to ensure the fluid was draining correctly. It is this fluid that causes extreme pressure in the brain and as a consequence, all-consuming agony – when your brain feels like it is pushing on the edges of your skull and the pounding is relentless. *Bam. Bam. Bam. Throbbing. Throbbing. Throbbing.* As though your brain is trying to hammer its way out of your head or escape, like an animal clawing at a cage that it's trapped inside.

My lesson that morning was with Mrs Wright, one of the most senior members of the school staff, a harsh and stuffy woman with a hollow, haggard face, short-cropped white hair and a long bony body. As soon as I entered the class, she reprimanded me for being late and told me to take a seat. At my desk, I lowered my tear-stained face and rested it on my crossed arms, hoping the migraine would ease off and the painkillers would kick in. But the pain and pressure only increased.

When I began to cry again, one of my friends asked if she could go into the cupboard and get my pillow. I had made it in textiles class: a blue pillow, decorated with a bright red cherry on the front. In the last few weeks, these headaches had become even more frequent and my friends knew I often put my head down on it during the breaks between lessons. This time, though, the pillow didn't help and I continued to cry. And I guess my sobbing had become audible.

'Michelle, I am finding it very hard to teach when you are being so loud,' Mrs Wright said. 'Can you keep it down?'

When I wasn't able to be quiet enough, she ordered me to leave the classroom. I stood, following her orders. I suddenly felt weak and unstable. I walked as far as the door and opened it, when I felt all the energy drain out of my body. I collapsed on the floor – just at the threshold between hallway and classroom – and lost consciousness for a split second, then awoke feeling out of focus and confused. I could feel the carpet burn on my face. Some of the girls in the class were screaming.

'She is going to be fine,' Mrs Wright announced in a deadpan voice. I remember thinking, even then, that her blasé-detached manner was very strange. 'She's just being a drama queen. Michelle, stand up, stop being silly. This isn't funny.'

Was I being a drama queen? Every time I had complained, cried and caused my parents to worry over the years, I had elaborately and carefully weighed the risk of that. I hated asking for special treatment. I hated making anybody worry. Ever since I could remember, people had been anxious around me, fretting and worried. As a baby I was listless, unable to sit up, and never learned to crawl. There was very little known about hydrocephalus in Hong Kong, where my family lived, and the doctors were largely inexperienced in how to solve it. The usual treatment is to instal shunts or, as I called them in my childlike language, 'tubes', which drain the water from the brain to the stomach. In Hong Kong, however, these tubes were installed in my body incorrectly and resulted in infections and blood poisoning – and left a latticework of surgical scars that cross my stomach and head. The drugs weren't much better. At the hospital in Hong Kong I got the nickname Barney, after the children's TV character, because whenever the doctors tried a new drug on me I turned purple. Eventually my parents flew me to Los Angeles, where a neurosurgeon at UCLA properly diagnosed and treated me, with even more surgery – partly to fix the bad work that had been done before. By the time I was seven, seven different surgeries had taken their toll on my body.

'Michelle. Please stand up.'

I managed to mutter only two words: 'I can't.'

Mrs Wright continued to speak to me as if I was capable of replying, as if this entire fainting episode was a game that I was playing and she was determined to make me lose.

'Well, at least turn over and move out of the door,' she continued. 'You are eating into valuable time with the class. Do you want to be selfish?'

My foot was propping the door open, and this uncertain position – not open, not closed – seemed to frustrate Mrs Wright as much as my motionless self on the floor.

'You are blocking the door, Michelle. I am only going to say this one more time. Stand up and stop making a scene.' She punctuated each word as if it were the end of a sentence, in equal parts venomous and eloquent, spoken in a slightly hushed tone so as not to cause a scene herself.

I remained silent.

'Michelle, this is your final warning. If you don't move, I will move you.'

Without a moment's hesitation, she walked over, bent down, took my head in her hands and moved it to the side, flipped the rest of my body over with her foot, and then tucked her hands under my arms and dragged me out the door and dumped me in the main foyer of the building – the exquisitely lovely arts centre of St Keyes: just one of many castle-like edifices on the extensive grounds of the esteemed school complete with lake, white swans and gloriously gloomy chapel. All the loving care and nonstop fundraising that had gone into maintaining its perfection, and the unassailable academic reputation of the school, was far from my thoughts as I felt only the carpet burns on my face and the frustration of not being able to speak or articulate how I was feeling.

I remember what I was thinking, though. *This is what it feels like to be dead. Or worse, to be lifted up like trash and placed on the side of the pavement.*

I rolled onto my side, the only position that had the potential of relieving some of the throbbing in my head, and wrapped my arms around my face tightly to block the glaring light and buffer the noise. I heard Mrs Wright on the classroom phone, making a call to the nurse. Then the school bell rang and my schoolmates began pouring into the corridor; some of them just walking around me, others stopping to see how I was.

'Everyone back in your classrooms now!' Mrs Wright bellowed. 'You are not to come out – stay inside!'

I opened my eyes briefly to see the expression on a girl's face who was asking for permission to go to the loo before her next lesson. The girl looked down at me woefully, with great pity. It was a look that I was accustomed to, but had gone to great lengths in my childhood to avoid. I closed my eyes to avoid her stare.

'Fine, but be quick!' Mrs Wright said impatiently. She walked around me and then knelt down in front of me, sending a strong waft of her pungent perfume in my direction. 'Look,' she said, lowering her voice to talk only to me, 'I realize you don't want to take exams and that you think faking it is the solution, but none of us are buying into this. These dramatic scenes will not be an excuse for you to miss your exams.'

### Trust.

'I'm not faking,' I stuttered. There was much more I wanted to say, but I was too fragile to utter another word.

'Look,' she continued, 'you won't get in trouble if you admit to us now that you are making this up, but if you continue – and we inevitably find out that you've been faking – you are going to be in serious trouble, Michelle.'

### Encouragement.

It wasn't just Mrs Wright who wanted this admission. If a guilty confession would've resulted in the relief of the excruciating pain, the words would've flown out of my mouth faster than I could think them. There was nothing I wanted more than to jump up and reveal this was all a joke.

Mrs Wright continued her inquisition, which was beginning to seem like a tactic used on prisoners of war and hardened criminals to get them to talk. 'Well, if you are so ill, then I am guessing you will have to stay in bed for all of half-term. What were you planning to do during half-term?'

Half-term at our school fell directly after our yearly exams. For that week, I had planned to go to France with my new best friend Annabel and her family. Annabel was a funny, outgoing, bright girl who was well liked by the whole year and our burgeoning friendship had helped me make the socially lonely transition to a new school. Annabel had an uncompetitive and open nature that was rare at St Keyes, where I was beginning to learn that relationships were fleeting and girls were quick to bad-mouth each other in an attempt to gain popularity.

As soon as I revealed my plans to Mrs Wright – 'I'm going to France with Annabel and her family' – I realized it was a mistake. This information gave her an edge, something she was hoping for.

'But if you are so, so ill, Michelle, surely you won't be able to make that trip. Which class is Annabel in? I am going to get her mother's number now and tell her that you can't make it.'

## Mutual Respect.

Unwittingly, Mrs Wright had gotten to the core of why I hadn't told my parents about the growing severity of my headaches over the year. I wanted a normal year and to have fun half-term plans like a normal girl. Usually, I told my parents everything. When I was sad, angry or emotional in any way, my dad was always my first call. He would listen carefully, give me good advice and calm me down. But I never talked to him about my health. Although we never spoke about this at home, many years before I was born, my dad had lost his first child, a seven-year-old boy named Michael, due to a fluke overdose of potassium in a Hong Kong hospital. This silently, yet dramatically, underscored my situation. Even more so because I felt my name was reminiscent of his, and emphasised the connection more than my sister or brother's names did. I never wanted to share anything that might cause my dad to worry. He had already gone through enough. Further to this, I knew that any discussion of pain would result in more tests, more doctor's appointments and at the very worst, hospital. A place which I was determined to never return to again.

Mrs Wright had a mobile phone in her hand. 'I'm calling Annabel's mother now…'

In that instant, two nurses arrived and helped lift me to my feet and walk me slowly to my dorm, at the furthest end of the school. The second that I was put in a bed, my head sunk into a pillow and my pain began to lessen – but did not ever go away. Three days later I was moved to the school's medical centre, where I spent four more days in agonizing pain, unable to eat, unable to keep anything down, drifting in and out of consciousness.

Mum arrived. That's the next thing I remember. The moment I saw her face, all the fear I had been suppressing came out in an overflow of tears. As I hugged her, I finally allowed myself to feel scared and worried. I had wanted to admit to my parents all I had been through, but didn't want them to fly across the world on my account. But her arrival meant I didn't have to ask. She came anyway. I knew she would look after me, make all the decisions for me, and advocate for my best interests. Being with Mum allowed me to be a child again, relieved of the burden of trying to assess and judge my symptoms or keep my headaches a secret. No longer would I have to be strong and pretend I was OK.

The nurses began packing up my clothes and belongings, while Mum helped me out of bed for the first time in days. As soon as I sat up, with my legs swinging down off the bed, a sharp pain hit me again. Mum helped me walk out of the school gates and get into the taxi, when the teacher accompanying my mum around the school called out in a chirpy voice, 'See you on Monday!'

That was just two days away. Would I really be better by then?

As I lay in the back of the taxi, with my head propped on Mum's lap, I drifted off to sleep and only awoke the following morning in my parents' bed at their London apartment. This was an indication of how sick Mum thought I was. Ever since I was little, probably like most children, there was something very special and comforting about being allowed to rest in my parents' bed. But it only happened when I was severely ill.

I looked around the room for my mum, but she wasn't there. Something else was missing too: no migraine. Perhaps all I had needed was a proper night's sleep in my own bed. *Maybe I was going to be OK*. This felt comforting until another thought occurred to me: it might have been stress from exams, or just my imagination, after all. It would be hard to prove I hadn't faked the whole thing.

I might have to return to school and issue an apology to the hideous Mrs Wright.

I decided to sit up – a physical movement that would cause the fluid pressure in my head to change. If I were truly unwell, the pain would return. I slowly placed my hands on the bed, propping my frail body against the head-board, and with a bang, the migraine returned – and with it, a mix of emotions.

Mum entered the room with a bowl of her homemade soup for breakfast. This provided me with brief solace until I noticed – and it wasn't difficult – that she had worried herself into a mode that was all too familiar to me: hysteria. She paced all over the room, then finally sat down long enough to become immersed in her laptop, and I knew her mind would be racing with questions and solutions. Mum had a fiery and passionate nature, and rarely sat still – something I assumed was the result of her upbringing in Singapore by Chinese parents, which had been Cinderella-like and harsh, full of hard work and the responsibility of raising her siblings. Right now, I attempted to stop her from making rash decisions, reassuring her that this was a passing phase, that I would be fine soon.

But I could see that it wasn't open for discussion. When my mum had her mind set, there was nothing to be done to change it. She was immoveable and headstrong. And despite her insistence that women be 'ladylike' and 'compliant' – something that was clearly drummed into her by her parents and culture – she was outspoken and non-compliant herself, particularly when she swung into

Mother Protectress mode. Well known among her friends as a 'character', she was actually quite a homebody and didn't like to socialize, yet when she organized the occasional dinner party for our near and dear, she went above and beyond. This was her way of expressing deep love and loyalty, along with home-cooked meals, carpooling and overseeing every aspect of my care and my brother's.

For Mum, love was demonstrated in deeds, not words. But in the last few months I had needed more reassurance. Over the Christmas break, my family and I had been stuck on a boat during the terrible tsunami in Thailand. When we came ashore, after the storm surge was over, we'd seen dead bodies on the muddy roadsides and heard the wails of grieving family members. Mum had told my brother and me to close our eyes – and not watch. But soon after, when I got back to school in England, I began insisting that each conversation with my parents end with the words 'I love you.' If we forgot to say it, I would call them back. This obsessive need for love to be conveyed, and not just shown, was met with confusion by Mum, who had grown up in a practical Chinese culture where children were born, and seen, only as eventual caretakers. She was a source of strength, a pillar of fortitude, and rarely displayed emotion or focused on her own needs. We were her priority. To her way of thinking, every action exuded love and words were just words.

'Why do you need me to say it again? Of course I love you. *Isn't it obvious?*' she would say, unnerved. 'My own mum has never told me that she loves me and I already told you yesterday I love you, so why would today be any different?'

Now, as I sat ruminating in her bed, Mum phoned local hospitals and called my dad back in Hong Kong, to discuss options. It was decided that we needed to fly to Los Angeles, where all my medical files were kept from my last surgery, as well as the neurosurgeon who had properly diagnosed and treated me when I was a little over one year old and then again when I was seven. Los Angeles? This seemed so extreme and sudden.

'We don't have time to waste,' my mum adamantly stated. In less than an hour, I was in the back of another taxi, my head resting on her lap. We were on the way to the airport. Except, in order to get on a flight to America, I needed to pretend that I was healthy. If I even looked vaguely ill, they wouldn't let me on board. Mum knew that better than anybody; before she married my dad, she had been a flight attendant.

At the airport I put on a smile and acted as though everything was OK – I was very good at that – but I still needed to take breaks to sit down regularly on our slow walk to the gate. On the plane, I rested my head on the cold window and fell asleep. After the flight attendants got word that I would be receiving medical attention upon arrival in Los Angeles, I was moved to an empty row of seats, where I was allowed to sleep lying down with a blanket and pillows. I woke from the bumps on landing. We had arrived.

# 2

## How did I end up back here?

Looking around the UCLA hospital parking lot, I felt uneasy and disorientated. My legs were shaking and unsteady. With a stumble, I scraped my knee on the cold concrete before landing in my mum's arms. The next few minutes were a whirlwind of people around me. I was lifted onto a gurney and wheeled into the hospital.

'You remember Dr Alfiderez?' my mum asked.

I struggled to recognize his face. 'Where is Dr Bentley?' He was the one I remembered and was used to.

The bright lights of the emergency room aggravated my headache. I curled onto my side and assumed my usual position – tucking my face between my arms to shield my eyes from the lights and buffer my ears from the sounds. My gurney kept moving, the rotation of its wheels softly reverberating through my body as I was rolled along passageways and never-ending corridors.

When I allowed myself to peek out into the world, the chaos of the emergency room terrified me – I felt a sense of true terror and panic. There had been a terrible shooting on the Los Angeles freeway and the wounded victims were all around me. Their blood was splattered on the walls and floors, in swirls and drips. Arguments and drunken conversations erupted in front of me, dramatic and charged, as if taking place in an action film with a scary twist – the kind of movies I was never allowed to watch. The nurses tried to protect me from views of the vomiting, urination and defecation, all of which filled the air with awful smells that made me wince and gag; I had to force myself to keep control over my own bodily fluids.

I focused on the cold, sterile hospital environment, familiar to me from the past – where people rush around you, poking and prodding and acting as if the human inside you no longer exists. I was lying on the gurney as hospital charts were passed over my head. I was handed off from one nurse to another, my gurney swapped again and again before being pushed through new corridors. I fell into my passive hospital self, the old hand who knew if she heard the words 'CT' or 'MRI', that it meant I would be heading to the jail cell of the imaging room. The walls would close in and I would feel very alone.

As a little girl, MRI scans and CT machines were a familiar part of my childhood, like medical check-ups and the scheduled doctor's appointments; but they never got easier and I always pleaded to have my mum by my side. Occasionally, if I made a big enough fuss, she would be allowed to stay with me. She would hold my foot, softly, gently, so I could feel her presence. But, most of the time, it was just me and a machine. The MRI was a perfect torture device; a place where I was paralysed both literally and figuratively, left alone with thoughts that I didn't want to have. The head brace was only a few inches from my face, escalating the sense of claustrophobia as the machine surrounded me and spun around my head. A voice inside kept saying, *Don't move. Don't move. Whatever you do, don't move.* If I did move, the scan would take twice as long. The noise of the machine provided the ideal sound-track for this isolation: a loud groaning and droning that circled and circled.

*How did I end up back here?*

The scans arrived quickly. They showed that nothing was amiss. That was when I began pleading quietly and silently for something to be wrong – otherwise my complaints had brought my mum all the way from Hong Kong to England and on to Los Angeles just for a simple headache.

As I lay on my gurney in the waiting room, I saw my mum in the far corner having a discussion with the doctor.

When they were finished, I was told that a procedure was going to take place. They were going to operate *just in case*. And they were going to operate *now*. Another emotional rollercoaster ride was beginning.

I hugged Pogo, my stuffed toy that Mum had given me which I'd brought from school to keep me company. I said goodbye to Mum and tried not to see the fear in her eyes, knowing she would be left to wait alone for the next couple of hours, and I nuzzled my head into Pogo's soft face. My gurney was rolled down more corridors and hallways. I felt a cool breeze against my robe as the door to the operating room was swung open. In the last four years of no-surgeries, I had forgotten this feeling – doctors and nurses surrounding me on either side, lowering the handlebars of my bed, lifting the sheet up from below, carrying me over to the metal plank where the operation would take place. I looked up at the lamps glaring in my face and the machines that were supposed to keep me alive. My breath quickened, a nervousness growing, an urge to get up and run out of the room, while they prepared the injection to put me under, and then the mask to follow.

Somewhere far away, in the foggy distance, I could hear voices counting down from ten, while my body became heavier and heavier and my mind slipped into nothingness.

Pain everywhere. A dull ache filled my entire body, weighing down on me as I struggled to open my eyes. Slowly awakening in yet another hospital room, a nurse and my mum were at my bedside. Thankfully, my mum had made the right decision in taking me to hospital. My tube – the shunt draining fluid from my brain – had been broken. I had a vague feeling I knew what had caused it, but I had refrained from mentioning it. A few months before, while playing with my neighbour in Hong Kong – a toddler, not much older than two – he had punched me in the neck. I immediately began to feel a little lightheaded but had continued playing with him, insistent nothing was wrong. It was only a week later, when the doorbell rang and I turned to answer it, that I suddenly lost my vision for an instant. My first thought at that moment was that it had something to do with my tube. Maybe the punch had broken it. So I ran my finger along my neck, down the side of my tube, as I had been taught to do ('You'll know if it's broken, because you'll feel a break…'). But I felt nothing – no break. My little self-test turned out to be wrong.

'How is the pain?' the nurses asked me.

Agonizing. But I wasn't going to share this in the presence of my mum. I could see panic in her eyes and exhaustion on her face. She had clearly been awake throughout the night as she awaited the news of my surgery.

I smiled to reassure her.

'Get some rest, Mum,' I said. 'I'm going back to sleep.'

Sleep was the easy solution.


Abdominal surgeries are dreadful to recover from. When they cut into your intercostal muscles, you become aware of how often you use them – for sitting up, standing, walking, reaching, and coughing. The worst was sneezing. When I cried out, the nurse urged me not to move and arranged the pillows around me.

Each day in the intensive care unit, I was assigned a new challenge, a new pain-inducing exercise to accomplish, from sitting up to walking. My main motivation was the goal of being able to use the toilet – rather than the soul-destroying process of having to relieve my bladder in a bedpan, and having my mother lift my bottom to insert the bedpan under me. I had never learned to aim properly, and bedding always needed to be changed. And the changing of the bedding only induced more pain, as I was rolled from side to side with three people holding my body in place. Eventually, after five long days, I made it to the toilet myself.

In celebration of this accomplishment, I was allowed to leave the hospital. Mum and I moved across the road, into short-term accommodation used by parents of young patients, where my mum had been staying all along. My dad was still in Hong Kong, looking after my brother who still lived back there.

Daily check-ups continued, as well as appointments and blood tests, but the freedom to walk outside and to eat something besides hospital food was a luxury that I promised myself I would never take for granted again.

On the day of my flight back to England – and back to St Keyes – Mum and I had a few hours to spare and we ventured a bit further into the city. Mum said we could do as much shopping as my body could handle. When was the last time anybody said this to you? I was excited beyond belief and quickly began searching for presents to give my friends and classmates, and a few things for myself.

We were in Los Angeles after all. And as we perused the shops, and settled into lunch, I found my stamina and strength returning.

Suddenly, it occurred to me that only a week had gone by since we left England. Hard to believe, but exams had just finished at school. This meant that my trip with Annabel was still a possibility – and I immediately began telling Mum about everything Annabel and I had planned to do in France, and how much I still wanted to go. Of course, Mum wasn't convinced. I had just had major surgery. Instead, she suggested that my dad come over from Hong Kong to England with my brother and we could spend half-term together in a calm, relaxing way. We began to bicker about this, just as lunch drew to a close. Frustrated, Mum stood up. It was time to leave. Just as I pushed out my chair and stood up, I began to sway and wobble. I caught a grip on the edge of the lunch table to keep myself from falling.

'Mum, I have something to tell you.'

She turned around and faced me. As reluctant as I was to say anything, I knew the moment for total honesty had come. And besides, here we were, in Los Angeles, where everything could be examined and properly studied.

'I have a headache.'

# 3

## Is my body even mine?

My mum and I walked down a long corridor of doors, identical except for the complicated arrangement of words on the front of each one, describing various medical specialties that made no sense to my eleven-year-old brain. Eventually we came to Dr Alfiderez's small office, its walls filled with thank-you cards from patients and academic certificates, each one reassuring me of his capabilities. Dr Alfiderez greeted us – a cheerful man with a gentle smile – and offered us a seat.

Like so many medical conversations, most of what he said was incomprehensible to me. It was mostly meant for my mum. Afterwards, he attempted to explain things to me, diluting and distilling the details to convey only the necessary information. Even so, it was a jumble of sounds and the doctor's accompanying drawings, which were meant to help, really didn't. They seemed like nonsensical doodles.

His drawing of the human heart was unrecognizable from what I thought hearts looked like. This only added to my confusion. Why was my heart was being discussed in the first place?

I began to zone out of the conversation, distracted by his array of thank-you cards, when I heard one sentence:

'We need to do it now,' Dr Alfiderez said to Mum. 'If the water causes the brain to sag any more, she may become paralysed. Her brain is already lower than it should be, and it could weigh on the spinal cord.'

Paralysis? This was new. I knew what this word meant from previous experiences in the hospital as a little girl. Being in close proximity to paralysed children was always sobering, a reminder that despite my complex conditions, my ability to move was one that I could be grateful for. And that my body, despite all its flaws, still kept me alive.

· It occurred to me – and bothered me – that in all the multitude of scans of my head that had been taken throughout my childhood, and recently, the position of my brain had never been described as 'low'.

Couldn't they build a shelf inside my head to stop it from sagging?

'Why has no one ever told me my brain was sagging?' I cried out, suddenly. 'You've operated enough times – why haven't you moved my brain upwards to stop it sagging? *I can't be fucking paralysed!*'

Mum gasped. 'Where on earth did you learn that word!'

'Mum, we have bigger worries than me swearing right now.'

'Don't swear!' she continued. 'It's not ladylike!'

*Ladylike?* Having been brought up in a culture where being docile and gentle was paramount to being feminine, my mum often found me lacking in this regard – despite her own headstrong nature. It was one of many battles that I'd had with her throughout my childhood.

Was being ladylike really important in the context of such a life-altering conversation? Over the years our arguments had grown in both volume and number, often leaving my father in the position of having to be the peacemaker. He was always calm and collected, in contrast to Mum's hotheadedness.

Nothing had ever made me as mad as this sagging brain conversation, though. The news radicalized me. I badgered Dr Alfiderez with questions, interrupting him and my mum repeatedly as they fumbled to find answers. Eventually I was ushered out of the room to avoid being further upset and causing myself 'unnecessary worry'.

With the slam of the doctor's office door behind me, a nurse appeared, as if by magic, and persuaded me to have another MRI scan. It was while I was lying in that awful empty chamber again that I began to see how little in my life I could actually control. All I had done was confess that I had a headache, and then, when the doctor had nudged me, that I had four or five of them a week, sometimes more.

'But that's not supposed to happen,' he'd said. 'That's not normal.' This led to the sagging brain explanation, the mention of paralysis... and just as I'd tried to deal with this revelation, I was removed from all decision-making and any further critical information was kept from me.

It was an effort to spare me the pain, but also the truth. The doctor and Mum shifted immediately into the PG, child-friendly version of what was going to happen to me. Shunts would be called tubes, migraines would be euphemized to headaches, and every gory and unpleasant detail would be wiped away to twist the true nature of events into an exciting new adventure.

I was told that a positive attitude was everything. I knew instinctively that I had to play along, because fighting, crying and objecting had no place in a 'serious situation'.

There was no choice, no control. I had to give up.

The MRI was followed by another visit with Dr Alfiderez. 'There is too much water in your head,' he said in a gentle voice, 'so we are going to put a metal valve around your tube to control it.'

He demonstrated how the valve would work, his hand encasing a straw, which served as a model of my tube. His hand squeezed the straw tighter, showing how the valve would control the flow of water from my brain. When I needed less water, the valve would tighten. When I needed more, it would open wider, which Dr Alfiderez demonstrated by relaxing his grip.

Then he dropped another bomb. 'There are also a number of tubes still in your tummy from your last operations,' he said, 'so we thought we would go in and tidy things up in there.'

*Was there a part of my body that* didn't *need surgery?*

To be perfectly honest, what bothered me most at this point was missing out on the trip to France. There I was, just hours from getting on the plane to London, having almost convinced Mum that I was well enough to take a holiday with Annabel, and then due to my own stupidity in confessing another headache, I was stuck in California, stuck at the hospital, and facing another surgery.

I tried to take it all back.

'But I don't even have a headache any more. It's totally gone. Isn't that weird? Must've been a passing thing. See – told you there was nothing to worry about.'

Despite all the drama classes that I'd taken as a girl, I wasn't exactly an award-winning actress. This scene convinced nobody. I began to cry as I started to think about another recovery process. I had just gone through one that was painful and excruciating. I had just gotten to the point where the pain across my stomach wasn't constant. To go backwards, and return to the land of pain, felt cruel. Realizing this, I was seized with a sudden resistance.

'I'm not doing it. I won't! I can't! No!'

Both Dr Alfiderez and my mum cajoled me. It was just a simple procedure, they said, and afterwards I wouldn't have headaches any more and everything could go back to 'normal'. After eight surgeries now, and eleven years of living with pain, I didn't believe them.

The recovery time would be only three days, Dr Alfiderez told me. I would be home in time to enjoy my half-term in England.

'Three days? You promise?'

'Three days. That's a promise.'

Everyone but me knew the truth: nobody recovers from brain surgery in three days. Their lies were supposed to help me muster the courage to face the operating room again.

Three days...

*I guess I could do that.*

But a piece of metal was being put in my brain? Dr Alfiderez assured me that only a quarter of my hair would be shaved in preparation for surgery.

'What? Don't you dare!' I cried out before I could control myself. 'You are going to have to leave me looking normal, otherwise you aren't doing it.'

His voice was inordinately calm. 'Michelle, this is important. The hair will be shaved near the bottom of your hairline, where it will be easily hidden. And besides, you are so beautiful, a bit of missing hair won't make a difference.'

'Leave a layer of hair to cover the stitches,' I bargained. 'I need to look normal. I am not going back to school looking like a freak with a half-shaved head. Otherwise, I refuse to have surgery.'

'OK,' he said. 'I am not a hairdresser but I will see what I can do.'

'I want a promise...'

Embarrassed, my mum interrupted. 'Michelle, stop this. It's good enough, Dr Alfiderez is very busy and all anybody can do is their best.'

You'd think my mum would understand – a shaved head is not ladylike, after all.

*

Before I knew it, with Pogo in hand, I was being wheeled into surgery again. Pogo kept me from facing what I knew to be true: that everybody goes into surgery alone. My mum would say goodbye, but Pogo was never taken from me.

The corridors were endless. My gurney rolled along, my charts were passed over my head, and I met one nurse after another, each of them using intimidatingly long words, and then, with the swing of the operating room door, a cold breeze hit my face. But this time, instead of the icy-white desolate room I was accustomed to, something was different. The operating room had fish and unicorns painted on the wall.

It was an operating room for children. It seemed horrific to me – and not a comfort. *All these sweet animals dancing on the wall of a room where children come to die.* A nurse asked me if I was OK in an overly positive manner, robotically, as if she had uttered the same sentence multiple times that hour already.

There was no correct answer, so I just mumbled, finding it hard to catch my breath because I was worrying so much.

'We look forward to welcoming you back in a couple of hours,' the nurse continued. 'For now, just relax.' She acted like I was simply boarding a plane, as if I was going to take a magical journey. More lies.

I closed my eyes.

I had never liked getting anaesthesia through a mask.

It made me feel like I was suffocating. So it had been a relief to be told I'd be having an injection instead.

But when I opened my eyes, a mask was quickly approaching my face.

I began to shake my head away, trying to refuse it.

'Don't worry,' the anaesthesiologist said. 'It smells really good – and tastes like bananas.'

I hated bananas. The mere whiff of banana smell had once actually made me vomit. It was the one food that could instantaneously induce a gag reflex in my throat. With my hands strapped to either side of me, like a prisoner, I angled my head away from the foul fruity smell.

A pair of hands held either side of my face, while another person placed the mask over my mouth. The smell of bananas enveloped me. I cannot begin to describe how truly sickening this was. Feeling more and more suffocated, I began to breathe faster and faster.

'Breathe slowly,' a voice said.

I wanted to fight it but the gas had already affected me. I began my usual mantra of happy thoughts, making myself think of *unicorns and fairies, unicorns and fairies, let's think about a princess...*

Thinking positive things just before surgery would keep me alive, or so I believed. Although I could never factually prove it, and never tested *not* doing it, I was convinced my faith in happy thoughts had worked for me all those other times. And it gave me something to do as I drifted off. It was certainly better than thinking about the pain I would have when I woke up, or how much I really wanted my mum, or my dad, whom I hadn't seen in two months.

Princesses, unicorns, fairies... Many times in my life since, my friends have told me I live in a fairytale world – that I am overly trusting and positive, to the point of being gullible. And perhaps this is why. Rather than an ordinary childhood in which I could dream about Prince Charming or luxuriate in a fear of boys giving me lurgies, I got this. Hospitals. Masks being put over my face. Tubes and needles. But there's a miraculous benefit to having to face adversity: you learn how to believe whatever you want to believe. The childhood that I created for myself was sweet and cartoonish. I wanted that so badly – and held onto that dream tightly until it became real.

Waking up in the children's intensive care ward, I had the familiar feeling of grogginess. Looking over, I saw my mum asleep next to me.

Everyone used to say I was so strong. Well, it wasn't me – it was my parents. How much easier their life would have been if I'd never been born. It was hard to wallow in self-pity when I thought about all the stress they'd been through. And my brother – how much happier he would be if I hadn't come along when he was less than a year old and sucked up all the family's energy and attention with my ongoing medical problems. Or even my sister, technically my half-sister, my dad's daughter from a previous marriage, had I taken away the attention from her too? If anyone in my family was suffering, I would willingly take away all their pain in an instant, but I couldn't. Instead, I was the one inflicting it.

My dry throat started to itch as I wheezed. I asked the nurse for water, awakening Mum.

'Are you OK?' she asked immediately, then launched into rapid-fire questions.

'How are you doing? Are you in pain? *Do you need anything?*'

I turned to look at her and felt a wound at the back of my head, a sensation I had never felt before. There was stinging, combined with the prickling of the stitches, surrounded by a dull ache that made it hard to think or keep one train of thought going. The pit of my stomach began filling with dread as I wondered how much of my hair had been shaved off. I was still drowsy, still under the influence of the anaesthesia, nodding in and out. Hours merged together. The lack of external light or access to a window, or view to the outside, warped my perception of time. I was not allowed to eat. As I woke up, I felt myself growing weaker and weaker. My mum was in a reverse gear: as I grew more tired, she moved faster and faster around me, becoming more persistent in her inquiries about my welfare.

Mum had a habit of hovering, micromanaging my care, often nitpicking about things she saw in my chart or something the nurses were doing. She reached her peak of anxiety immediately after surgery. She ran around making trouble for everybody. Talking, questioning. My hospital bed was separated from the beds of other patients by only a thin sheet hanging from a rod near the ceiling. I tried in vain to calm her down and get her to relax. 'Mum, stop! People are trying to sleep! You're disturbing everyone on the ward!'

A chorus of heart-rate monitors and the beeping of other equipment combined to form an annoying hospital symphony around me. From the sounds alone, I guessed there were roughly ten people in the room with me, each patient as critically ill as the next.

It was impossible not to be embarrassed by the way my mum was hogging the nurse's time with her questions and second-guessing, preventing her from properly attending the other patients. She trapped the poor nurse in the corner, and then they walked over to my bed.

'See how her stomach is inflamed?' my mum was saying, lifting the sheet and gesturing towards my stomach. 'This isn't normal.' She talked over me, completely unaware of the fact I was trying to speak. All her attention was on my abdomen. An additional procedure had been done – vaguely mentioned the day before. An incision had been made in my stomach in order to remove the old tubes that weren't being used any more. This would mean much, much more pain to come, and not just in my head.

'Mrs Elman,' the nurse responded, 'this is completely normal post-surgery. The swelling will go down in a couple of hours. You don't need to worry. You must be tired. The best thing would be to go home and rest.'

I urged my mum to follow the nurse's instructions, but she wouldn't let up. 'I want her doctor on the phone right now,' she persisted. 'Either you take my daughter for a scan or you get him on the phone! I know something is wrong.'

This was the last thing I needed. No way in hell was I going for another scan, let alone an unnecessary one. Mum's basic over-protectiveness, escalated by anxiety, worry, sleep deprivation and low blood sugar, had become a perfect storm of paranoia.

My level of embarrassment – at least nine or ten patients on the other side of the curtain drawn around me were witnessing this diatribe – was at an all-time childhood high.

'Mrs Elman,' the nurse said, her voice becoming sharper, 'it is three in the morning. Michelle's doctor is not in the hospital. He is asleep at home. And even if we sent her for another test, the waiting time for the CT scan will take at least two hours. How about we wait until the morning to see if the swelling has gone down?'

Mum only grew more irate. It wasn't until she stormed out of the room in a huff that I felt relief and had a moment of post-op peace in the solitude. It didn't last long. Half an hour later, I opened my eyes and saw Dr Alfiderez and my mum standing over my bed.

'Oh my god, Mum!' I cried out. 'You are so embarrassing! I'm so sorry, Dr Alfiderez – she's dragged you out of bed for nothing!'

Even if the nurses and doctors who were working so hard around me in the children's unit were accustomed to overbearing parents, I was still mortified by my mum's behaviour.

'Your mum was right to call me,' Dr Alfiderez intervened.

'Something *is* wrong, Michelle, and I'm afraid we are going to have to take you back into surgery. We are going to do a quick scan, which means you have to drink this contrast as soon as you can. Then you will head straight into surgery.'

Contrast is a kind of liquid dye that you swallow before a CT scan. That was bad enough, but wait – *another surgery? Could my mum have actually been right?*

Rather than fully comprehending the gravity of the word 'emergency', which was now being used around me, my focus went to this bottle of liquid: the contrast. It was the part of the MRI and CT ritual that I hated most. Throughout my childhood, I had been squeamish and fussy about unpleasant tastes, and often unable to keep the contrast down. But it was mandatory. Until I drank it, there would be no scan.

A bottle was handed to me. I looked down at the label. It said 'BANANA FLAVOUR'.

'You have to drink three bottles.'

As much as I was aware of the importance of drinking this liquid, I struggled. After every couple of gulps I would gag and the liquid would come back up into my throat and mouth. A tray was held under my mouth as I continued to drink and regurgitate, and things were going slowly. 'Can you not just inject it into me?' I asked.

Mum became impatient, her face contorting with a kind of fear that I had never seen in her before. I sensed another thing: a weird vibe in the people surrounding me, a hesitancy that I couldn't put my finger on, but one that strongly suggested that whatever was happening to me – whatever they were worried about – was a whole new level of serious.

Explanations were provided to help motivate me. The liquid was necessary to light up the areas of my body that needed to be studied, and made things clearer on the scan. I nodded. Facts can help. And did. I began to chug down the liquid, and when it resurfaced in my mouth, I was able to swallow it again. One bottle finished. Two more to go.

My mind switched into a new gear: survival mode.

*An emergency surgery, Michelle. This is important. Emergency. What don't you understand about that? Start drinking.*

I continued to mentally fight with myself, and began to vary my methods to keep this liquid down. I tried drinking quickly. I tried drinking slowly. I tried it with sugar. I tried while holding my nose. After an hour had past, my doctor came to see my scan and discovered that, because of the struggle to get the contrast down, I hadn't even had it yet.

'We will need to go into surgery now without it,' Dr Alfiderez said. Then he told my mother to call my father. 'He needs to be here, just in case.'

*Just in case.* I knew what that meant.

My dad hated flying. He was a nervous flyer. In fact, he'd been a passenger on a flight once when a flight attendant had tried to soothe his nerves by telling him it was her birthday. She confessed eventually that her birthday had actually been a few days before – which meant that she and my father had the same birthday. That led to a date, and later to marriage, and my brother and me.

And now this.

A nurse appeared with a form for Mum to read. 'You need to sign this before Michelle goes into surgery,' the nurse explained. 'It confirms that you will not sue for costs if she doesn't make it.'

My heart dropped. It's difficult to describe what I felt at that moment. Conflicted was the main thing. Worried for me. And even more worried for my mum. I didn't want her to be more scared than she had to be.

And I thought about my dad. People in the business world thought of him as serious and stern, but to me – and the rest of his family – he was compassionate, caring and funny. He never spoke when it wasn't necessary yet always exuded a sense of strength, even when silent. He understood people. And he had always understood me. In many ways, he was my closest friend and greatest ally in life.

I thought back to the last time I'd spoken to him. I'd been really tired from the last surgery and hadn't told him I loved him. I couldn't remember what the last sentence had been, but it wasn't 'I love you'. That really panicked me; my obsessive habit had been broken, and of all the times. Now I wanted to speak to him, just for a second. Just in case.

He always said, 'Call me anytime, 24/7/365. Day or night. It doesn't matter. I'm always just one phone call away.' Why hadn't I called him more?

They rolled me along the corridor and into the operating room, and transferred me onto the operating table. At that point I realized that I didn't have Pogo; everything had happened too quickly to remember him.

The nurses and technicians stopped making their polite small talk. I heard their voices rise and grow tense. Something wasn't right. 'Page him now,' I heard one of them say. 'Get him here now – quickly.'

The cold metal slab underneath my body felt colder. My racing heart felt like it was breaking the walls in my chest, it was beating so loudly. That's when it occurred to me that I actually might die. And what consumed me were thoughts of my parents. I had inflicted so much pain on them already, and now my mum was going to be counting down the uncertain minutes alone in the waiting room while my dad flew halfway across the world. After a twelve-hour flight, would he arrive in Los Angeles to learn that he had one less child? Again?

I was terrified… and the worst part: so was everyone else in the room. I felt a pinch in my arm, a slow warmth rising up my arm. I looked down to see the intravenous needle sticking out of my skin. I swam towards the warmth, towards sleep. And I remembered to fill my head with positive thoughts. *Princess. Fairies. Unicorns. You're good at this. Princess. Fairies. Unicorns. You've done this before.*

# 4

## Am I OK?

Noise. I heard people talking in the background, the familiar sounds of beeping and monitors and phones ringing in the distance, a rustle of papers near my ear and my mum talking to the nurse. And my dad. I heard his voice. Dad!

'When will she wake up? Will everything be OK? Will she be affected?'

My parents had just arrived in my room. I could tell by the questions they asked – the rushing to get all the answers immediately. I wanted to be a part of it. I wanted to say hello, to open my eyes. But instead I felt trapped inside my body. I couldn't feel my legs. Each breath was an effort, my chest was heavy, and each movement brought deep pain across my stomach. I could tell it had been a large incision this time. The harrowing pain indicated its severity. It was unlike anything I had ever felt before; as if they'd removed each of my organs and replaced them with sandbags.

*Please don't say they removed all my organs.*

There were so many new sensations. I could feel the pain around each coil of my intestine, and where my stomach supposedly lay was a dull ache, then with each breath a sharp pain, making me want to curl into a foetal position. I kept trying to open my eyes but the muscles in my eyelids weren't working. Both my parents continued to talk as if I wasn't there – meaning I heard things I wasn't supposed to.

I attempted to twitch my eyes. They felt stuck together, like the lids were glued shut, presumably due to some residue from my surgery. I tried to lift my hand and this required intense conscious thought. Upon trying a few times, the energy in my body couldn't manage it, and I began to cave into the temptation to go back to sleep. Then I felt a cool, wet cloth over my eyelids. The nurses had clearly got the hint from my twitching and wincing.

'Welcome back,' a voice said.

Then it occurred to me that I had survived. I was alive. I was breathing. But...

Am I OK?

Dad was there. That's what I remember most. He was looking at me. Even more than the joy I felt at seeing him, I remember the incredible relief of knowing that he hadn't flown across the ocean, all that way, to see another child die. His warm embrace eased my pain and having him there with my mum, together, brought me so much reassurance.

The surgery had taken eighteen hours. They'd had to fix something in my intestines because of a problem... Something else that had been done incorrectly.

Over the next couple of days I heard arguments back and forth – between my parents and the doctors. An inexperienced intern had made a mistake. UCLA is a teaching hospital, and the intern had been allowed to operate on me. To be fair to the intern, the attending physician on the case hadn't realized that due to my previous surgeries, I had what doctors called a 'frozen stomach'. My surgeries were therefore more complicated because my organs were wrapped in scar tissue – something like a jigsaw puzzle disguising what was underneath. *A kidney or a lung? You guessed wrong!*

The intern had punctured my intestines when pulling at one of the tubes. The other doctors hadn't noticed and sewed me back up, not realizing my intestines were leaking. An infection had spread, which meant that my shunt had to be removed and the remaining incision would need to be left open, in order for the infection to clear, for the next eight weeks. This explained the tremendous pain that I felt. They had cut right across my whole stomach, connecting two of my existing scars and cutting much deeper. And, because it was an emergency, they worked less carefully, resulting in a scar that was wider and much more prominent than my old one.

Covered up with a white bandage, what had been done to my stomach was yet to be revealed to me. It would be another few years before I'd see that this new scar would impact me for the rest of my life, creating a noticeable indent in my stomach that is visible even under a shirt. For now, though, my stomach was stapled open until the infection was clear. And I was moved to the children's intensive care unit, where I would remain for the foreseeable future.

My mum, in all her hysteria, had been right. A mother's instinct, I guess. She saved my life.

# 5

## Am I worried about dying?

The UCLA ICU (intensive care unit) is a cold, barren, efficient place. Everything exists for necessary purposes and anything else, anything decorative, is considered a hazard – a possible barrier that could undermine what is essential to help a patient in the event of an emergency. It is a large open-plan room where all the beds occupied by children are laid out in a circle around a nurses' station in the centre. Here, the moment when a life hangs in the balance is not an uncommon occurrence – a heart stopping, a last breath, the beeping of a monitor becoming flat and persistent, or a child bleeding out and being rushed on a gurney out of the room. Each patient is either critically ill or needing constant observation. It is much like the emergency room; chaos and crises are routine, almost on the verge of welcomed.

Every morning, before dawn, I was awakened during

rounds for an assessment. The thin sheet of curtain that lay between my bed and the nurses' station was drawn open and a group of young doctors would surround my bed while the white bandage that covered my entire abdomen was pulled off and my incision was drenched in a frigid-cold brown liquid. Iodine. This was used to clear the infection. Usually I would wake from the pain of stinging and a series of questions would follow – all mundane, not kindly or sensitively delivered – about my name and the date, to check that my brain function was fully intact.

What day of the week? This always struck me as peculiar, since I had no access to clocks or calendars or any other indicators of the passing of time, or even the ability to see the sun, moon or stars outside a window. The perception of days and months became warped and, despite my brain functionality being intact, the morning question about the date always puzzled me, much like when you're on school holidays and, without your regular schedule or the need to see a weekly planner, the days fade into each other.

For the majority of these assessments, while I would groan, I was otherwise compliant and responded to their queries. I kept my eyes closed in the hope that this would increase the likelihood of being able to fall back to sleep once they left, but this daily hope was dashed with the final test.

My eyelids were pried open and a torch was shone directly into my eyes.

I never understood what this tested, but it guaranteed that I would wake up figuratively on the wrong side of the bed every day. That, and the businesslike approach of the doctors, who were all students and without any bedside manner, started my day in a trying way. To them, I was a name on a chart. I was a body to study. As they discussed my condition, the most senior doctors would ask questions and the surrounding interns would fight to be allowed to respond. It was a demoralizing process, but even so, I was often thankful that they were talking about me and not to me. That was the last thing I wanted.

If I had a nice nurse, she would leave me in peace after the doctors had moved on, allowing me to sleep until my parents arrived during visiting hours. If not, it was time to give me a sponge bath and change my sheets. As I was unable to move, changing my sheets involved rolling me onto my side while they removed half the sheet and then rolling me back as they removed the other half. If the morning slathering of iodine or the bright flashlight beamed directly into my eyes hadn't been enough, this was sure to wake me up – as the rolling pulled on my abdominal muscles, which were weak and still healing, and forced the back of my head, where the incision was, to move on the pillow. This torture sequence left me feeling grumpy, groggy and sleep-deprived; a strange condition for someone who was living her life, day in and day out, in a bed.

A bit later in the morning, at 9 am, my favourite TV show, *The Bold and the Beautiful*, would come on. Watching this soap opera was one of the two highlights of my day, and a moment of continuity in my life. In Hong Kong, throughout my childhood, my mum and I would rush home from school and get our daily dose of the ongoing drama, and then binge-watch it on Sunday mornings. At boarding school I had missed this routine, but now I was fully immersed in it again, watching it intently. Soon after, the doctors would make another round, checking in to see if the infection was improving and then ordering any additional scans, injections or whatever was prescribed to be my daily dose of torment.

I would then nap on and off for the next two hours, until one of the 'play specialists' would arrive with a windmill to paint or some other arbitrary activity to fill up my day. There were quite a lot of windmills to paint. I found this most ironic. Where was the wind? Where was the sunlight? Once the thing was decorated, there was nothing whatsoever to do but use your own breath to make it spin.

The true highlight came at 3 pm. This was my second slot of TV time – and an important part of my pain relief. In the morning, *The Bold and the Beautiful* was there to help me with perspective and attitude. Whatever I felt, or whatever I'd been through, never seemed as awful as what was happening on the show, with its cast of characters who were either dying or involved in scandalous love affairs. The content wasn't always age-appropriate, but my innocent ears seemed to filter out those sections naturally, missing the occasional joke but enjoying the grown-up romance and intrigue of it all.

In the afternoon, *Full House* did the opposite: it helped me to recapture my innocence – something I dearly needed to cling to. For that half-hour, I didn't have operations,

I wasn't in a hospital, I didn't have a bed-ridden child-hood. I had joined the endearing household of the Tanner girls, three sisters growing up in a stereotypical way. They even had a character for me – Michelle, who became my favourite. She had this natural charm, something I so wished I could capture. Each of her catchphrases brought a smile to my face, even on the bleakest days. It was a slice of joy, my solace, and the very thing I felt I was living for.

Later in the afternoon, Uncle Cameron, my godfather, would come with his daughter, Julia. They lived in LA and visited me almost daily. Uncle Cameron and my dad had met at a dinner shortly before my birth and over the years had become exceptionally good friends – a modern-day bromance that was a beautiful thing to behold. Both my godfather and my godmother – my mum's best friend in Hong Kong whom I'd known since I was born – were important people in my life, and despite the traditional meaning of their titles they actually held no religious significance. Uncle Cameron was in the fashion business, and whenever he visited Hong Kong for work we became his second family. He brought out the youthful side of my dad, provoking a certain smile – cheeky, boyish, a little like my older brother's – that seemed to be reserved only for Uncle Cameron. At UCLA he became a nurses' favourite and was always filling my hospital bay with laughter. He and I had a very special relationship too; quick to tease each other with almost-too-snarky humour, yet generous with our hugs and kisses. His daughter Julia was a gentle soul, sensitive and compassionate like her dad, and much older than me – a proper adult at the age of twenty-three – but she fast became my friend. She was so effortlessly glamorous and lived a life I could only dream of one day having. She had a job at the Barbie doll company in Los Angeles and her gifts adorned my section of the ward, challenging its sterility and making it more welcoming. Along with her dad, she brought normality to my life. And unlike my parents, it was easy for them to be joyful and hide all signs of concern about my health. Their arrival didn't just lift my spirits, but it eased the stress for my parents whose constant attendance at my bedside was beginning to show its impact.

I hated the evening, when my parents were forced to leave at 7 pm, when a brigade of unhelpful night-shift nurses went on duty. Each night I fought the strict regimentation and pointless rules of the hospital, arguing that my parents should be allowed to stay over, or even just remain a few more hours. Whatever nurse was on duty would explain that if all parents were allowed to stay over, the result would be a very crowded and chaotic ward and a health and safety hazard for all the young patients. But how was this different from the ward during the day? And why had such an arbitrary time of 7 pm been chosen? The nurses never backed down. It was their job to enforce the rules, even if they made little sense. And eventually, just as I had in school, I grew bored with fighting the regime and to avoid the bleakness of the ICU at night, I tried to drift off to sleep as soon as possible.

How long would I be there? This was one question I

never asked, never wanted to know. I was afraid of the answer. But I held onto the fact that I was apparently getting better.

It was hard not to feel pangs of jealousy as I watched other children leave the ward to return home. The turnover in the ICU was faster than I had expected. I was the longest-standing patient there – in the same bed, next to the same wall, with the same visitors every day; and while my instinct was to be sad about the days and weeks that I was logging there, I also felt extremely grateful that I was still around, because some weren't.

I witnessed the passing of one small boy, not much older than ten, an experience that became etched in my brain and never forgotten. A sense of panic surrounded the boy's final moments as nurses rushed to his bedside and his parents were ushered to him. I remember the sound of his heart monitor, as it became one long continuous beep. His mother crumbled to the floor; her hysterical crying rose up and took over the room. The boy's father attempted to comfort her while inconsolable himself. The mood of the entire ward shifted palpably. An unbearable sadness spread across the room. Everyone walked with their bodies slightly hunched and their faces were solemn. No jokes were funny, and no bad behaviour was reprimanded – only acknowledged with a quiet nod. I grappled with the profound inequality of life, and its randomness. Who decided who lived and who died?

Maybe we all had a certain amount of luck and his had run out. Maybe I had a certain amount of luck – and it would run out soon too. Maybe this was a competition where only one of us would make it out alive. These things swirled around in my mind as I tried to make sense of it all. But there was no sense.

A weekly visit from a volunteer and her dog helped me to avoid descending into despair. I was still unable to sit up in bed, so this visit consisted of the dog lying near my head and me petting it for an hour. I'm not entirely sure why this had such a huge impact on me, but when Angel appeared and I was able to stroke her fur and study her brown, black and white patches, feelings of contentment and peace came over me. She was a large dog, and at first I worried that her weight would be too much for the bed and my body to bear, but then she rested her big head on my leg and I realized how gentle and sweet she was.

Angel reminded me of things in life I used to enjoy – when I was younger, back in Hong Kong, when I often spent the better part of the weekend walking my godmother's dogs and running around with them in her garden. Angel's visit was only one hour a week, but it was one hour of relief and peace. One time, when the nurses had other plans for me that conflicted with my hour with Angel, I cried so hysterically and so persistently – I was inconsolable – that it was feared my heart rate and blood pressure would be raised to an unhealthy extent. The sodium loss from crying was also something they were desperate to avoid. Don't cry, I was told. It could kill me.

Lying flat in bed, unable to walk or move around, I was also unable to wash my hair. The scar on my head needed to heal. A scab was forming over the skin graft and washing my hair would cause damage to it. Although it is true that eventually your hair ends up washing itself, this takes around a month to kick in. And it hadn't been a month yet. Up until this point, my hair had been so greasy that it often felt wet – oil-drenched and slippery. As if the half-shaved head didn't make me feel weird enough, having this slicked-back hair definitely ensured I didn't feel beautiful.

My scalp was incredibly itchy, too, and it was really hard to resist picking at my scabs, but a few bloody episodes had taught me to simply rub my head along the pillow when it itched, or gently run my fingers through my slick hair, which resulted in my hand being covered in grease. I got in the habit of wiping it on my duvet cover or bedsheet. Then, one day, when the tickling of my scalp reached a new level of awful, I stuck my fingers into my hair, massaged my head, and when I pulled it out, there was something crawling on my hand.

Two insects. Two head lice were on my fingers. I screamed in horror. The nurses rushed over and inspected my hair, and their faces began to show their disgust. Before I knew it, they had sectioned off my area with a neon yellow curtain and they'd changed into special robes and put masks on. Although nits are fairly common among schoolchildren, particularly in boarding schools, in the hospital they were considered extremely dangerous. A health hazard and safety concern. When the word 'contagious' was used, I was reminded of a recent storyline on *The Bold and the Beautiful* when one of the characters had tuberculosis. Her name was Taylor Hayes and she had contracted the disease while pregnant with twins. She was soft, kind and gentle – and most importantly, beautiful. A kind of beauty I envied. A type of beauty that didn't come with oil-slicked, nit-infested hair. Her mothering presence brought warmth to the show and provided a moral compass that was necessary in a world of drama, and her passionate and loving relationships echoed the fantasy of what I dreamed a relationship would be like. In my innocence, I found it exciting that I could be likened to that character.

'Cool!' I thought. 'It's like I have TB.'

Whether it was nits or tuberculosis, the response of the hospital was fairly similar: I was put in an isolated room and all medical personnel attending me had to wear protective gear. The doctors were also concerned that an infection could develop near the incision site on my head – and worried that my body might not be capable of fighting two infections at the same time. The nurses began combing through my hair every day to manually remove each louse. While I had been as alarmed as everyone else when the nits were first discovered, I soon found it very enjoyable to taunt visitors, and almost anyone in proximity, by pretending to throw nits in their direction. The upside of this childish prank: I was officially moved to the only private room in the entire ward. This room had its own TV and the incredible luxury of a door, allowing me privacy even if the door always had to remain open.

By this point in my stay, I had earned a reputation as a brat among the nurses. This had been conveyed to me via conversations with Rachel, the head nurse, while trying to persuade me to be a little less difficult. Rachel knew me from a previous stay at UCLA when I was little. She even appeared in the baby photo albums that my mum had made for me – the ones I had flipped through, over and over, almost obsessively. As a girl, I had stared at Rachel's blonde hair and captivating blue eyes, and never expected to see her again. But here she was, now the head nurse of my ward.

Apart from Rachel, there was only one other nurse with a particular fondness for me. Melissa was younger, a relentlessly happy and bubbly woman, recently engaged to be married. She rarely seemed tired or distracted; the wear and tear of her long twelve-hour shifts never showed. Well liked on the ward, and with the other patients, she might have been too popular to work only with me – except that, luckily, Rachel had created rotation schedules that allocated nurses to patients. Melissa became my friend and confidante in the absence of my parents, and her love for and dedication to her job made it feel special to be with her. Another plus: she laughed at my dark jokes and was amused by my rebellions.

We spent most days discussing the details of her upcoming wedding: how the veil would perfectly flow over her long red hair, how her dress would hug her curves perfectly, and which family guests were being invited. And on the days that I didn't want to talk, she would quietly keep me company. I learned a lot from this kind woman – most of all how important small gestures are in showing that you care. It was on one of these quieter days – a day when I was in a great deal of pain, hadn't been able to sleep and just wanted to be left alone to cry – that she popped down to the hospital shop and purchased a neon green-and-yellow beanbag toy frog and surprised me with it. This gesture was enough to finally dry my tears and bring a smile to my face. Melissa explained that it should help with sleeping because it was softer than the pillow. It wasn't the magic of the beanbag toy that worked; it was Melissa's kindness. It truly meant a lot to me that she had made the extra effort.

But her greatest gift was patience. As the weeks dragged on in the ICU, and then rolled into months, I became only more rebellious and difficult. The independence that had been nurtured, fostered and encouraged in boarding school had no outlet in this confined existence. My resentment grew, and my awareness of life's inequities and realities became more acute. Outbursts of emotion were the only release – usually a crying jag or an expression of attitude. I hated being patronized by the hospital staff and I was quick to retaliate if I felt belittled. Melissa never talked down to me or expected me to act like a nice, polite, lady-like eleven-year-old.

She had a name for my rebelliousness. She called it my 'sass'. And without encouraging it, she allowed me to relieve my boredom and desperation with unpopular pranks and inappropriate comments. These were varied but usually dark, often involving some element of playing dead or faking a severe impairment. One morning, I was beyond-irritated with the ritual of being awoken with the slathering of cold iodine on my stomach and the blindingly bright torch shone in my eyes. When I was asked by the attending doctor for the date and day of the week to ensure that my mental faculties were humming along, I replied with a date years in the past and watched with amusement as all the doctors began to whisper to each other in shock.

One doctor followed up with a question about my first name. I replied with my middle name, rather than saying 'Michelle', in order to escalate their worry. Melissa, who was overseeing this performance from the corner, remained quiet long enough to allow me some fun, then revealed to the doctors that I was just being 'Little Miss Mischievous'.

More harmless, but equally annoying, pranks were things like raising my hospital bed – it had a hydraulic lift – and enjoying the ability to touch the ceiling. Other times, I was content to play with my morphine drip, pressing it so that I'd be delivered excessive amounts of narcotics. This didn't go unnoticed. Eventually, the pain medication was given to me in injections so that I couldn't control my own dosage and the contents of my drip was swapped out to only contain water – although they never informed me of this. This meant that I often would press the button repeatedly with the belief that it was making me loopy on drugs. I began acting like it too, until Melissa mercifully told me the truth.

There were no playmates in the ICU. Children populated the beds but we were confined to them, hooked up to monitors, wires and tubes. Despite my desire for privacy, it was also becoming exceedingly difficult to exist without the company of my peers, having got used to the hustle and bustle of boarding school and the camaraderie in our mutual suffering. Surely hospital could be the same? Except here the suffering didn't come with humour, but instead the very real possibility of death. Curtains were pulled closed around us for privacy and with my new private room, I felt more isolated than ever. In the busy, chaotic room, we were lonely islands, and knew we were supposed to keep our thoughts and feelings to ourselves. We avoided interaction with each other. To be honest, it was a way to evade any more loss or sadness.

It was rare to know a child's name, or even see them up close. Melissa kept me informed about how her other patients were doing and provided me with updates. Although I couldn't move from my bed and could barely turn my head, it gave me relief to know that others were recovering, progressing and doing better. After witnessing that boy's death, I wished for no more moments of sadness and loss. But the walls of my private room were not thick enough to prevent overhearing the emergencies, the heart rate monitors dropping and in some cases flat-lining.

Even if I never saw them – or met them – I couldn't help but think about the other children nearby. When I heard sounds of other children in the ward, I feared the worst. I couldn't help but think of the opportunities that would be missed, the possibilities that had vanished, the milestones that would never be experienced, the relationships and emotions that would never be witnessed. At least in the geriatric wards the patients had their memories, but it seemed to me that here in the children's ICU was where dreams, idealism and naivety came to die.

Dreams were luxuries here; something reserved for healthy children. For those of us in the hospital, chronically ill, they were cruel taunts about a life that may never be lived. Few of us would have a future – or, at least, the future we had hoped for and dreamed about. We would always be limited by our disabilities, conditions, illnesses and scars. Even outside the hospital, for most of us, the worries and paranoia consumed us – and the fear of returning. This was our story. And it was always going to be our story. You could see it in our eyes and branded across our bodies. The scars were constant reminders that we would always be different. If you had the good fortune to leave the confines of the ICU permanently, you left a different person. You were no longer a child.

One of the smallest and youngest of my hospital-mates was a tiny baby named Meg Ryan. I remember her name because it was the same as the famous actress. She was only six months old and had been living all that time in the hospital, waiting for a heart transplant. Her parents came every day, without fail, and often carried Baby Meg around the ward, sometimes popping into my room to say hi and tell me how Baby Meg was doing. They would coo and gush with love as they held her, making her smile or laugh, and always remarking what a happy and delightful baby she was. Depending on how I was feeling that day, I would either be jealous that she was too young to comprehend her miserable situation, or I would feel guilty. Here I was, complaining about my confinement when this little baby had never been outside the walls of the hospital.

Illness is the greatest equalizer in life. It doesn't discriminate between the old or the young, the rich or the poor, the good or the bad, the kind or the selfish. Regardless of how good your life is, how much success you've achieved, all of it means nothing when you're in hospital. We were all equals there, in the same robes, in the same beds, separated by the same blue paper curtains. Even when it came to my private room, it was not given to me as a reward for my morality or for monetary reasons but instead an allocation chosen out of necessity to protect the other patients from my contagiousness. Visitors came to see me, each person trying to comfort me with stereotypical phrases such as 'everything happens for a reason' and the like. With each repetition of this phrase, I began questioning what the reason was. What had I done to deserve this? Increasingly, my life was beginning to seem like a cruel version of survival-of-the-fittest, a weeding out of the weak. How strong was I?

All these emotions began to create conflicts within me. I heard a heart monitor signalling another death, and I struggled with dark feelings – fear and guilt. Most people don't feel they have to earn a right to live, and certainly not most eleven-year-olds, but after witnessing so many emergencies and deaths, I began to feel that I was participating in a morbid competition. We were all on death row, and some of us were going to outlast the others. What had I done that was so valuable to earn the right to live?

Other days I was full of anger, as I noticed that some children were progressing and moving on to less serious wards. People tried to keep me upbeat, telling me to be grateful and that this whole experience would make me stronger and more appreciative of what I had before. Phrases like 'you're lucky, you have the best care in the world' were used so often that they may as well have recorded a track, almost like a propaganda machine of positive thinking, and piped it into my room through speakers. I hated it, and hated all attempts to cheer me up. It didn't feel encouraging; it felt like a demand that I try to be happy. My frustration about this would routinely send me into a rage and I would yell everyone out of my room. If I thought about school, or was asked about it, I became even angrier. In those days prior to easy wi-fi and social media, I had heard nothing from St Keyes or my classmates there. Summer term would soon be drawing to a close and the likelihood that I would still be in hospital was growing. And the angrier

I would get, the more positive everyone around me would become – often only making things worse.

About three months into my stay in the ICU, one day while I was watching *Full House* a woman walked into my room. She didn't seem to be a nurse. She didn't wear the scrubs like the nurses or the white coat like the doctor but had a badge that hung around her neck, indicating she worked in the hospital.

She began talking to me. Since I was fully engrossed in my show, I paid no attention to her. I didn't even raise my eyes from the screen to look at her and to this day I couldn't tell you what she looked like.

'Michelle, can you hear me?' she asked in a frustrated voice. 'I am trying to talk to you.'

Melissa was nearby and stepped in, explaining to the woman that I was watching one of my favourite TV programmes and could she wait another fifteen minutes until the break?

The woman replied that she had scheduled this time to meet with me. And I appeared to be free. What was the problem? She didn't understand.

'Yes,' Melissa explained, 'but when you're eleven years old and confined to your bed with nothing to keep you occupied except two half-hour television shows, plus a weekly session with a dog, these minutes become sacred.'

From my perspective, the woman had appeared at exactly the wrong time.

The woman didn't agree. She took the TV remote from the table and switched the power off.

'Michelle,' she said, 'I've come here to talk to you because people are growing concerned about your wellbeing.'

'Give me back the remote and come back in twenty minutes,' I said, defiantly.

'No, Michelle. I am here to talk to you now. I am not coming back later. I want to ask you how you are feeling.'

*How was I feeling?* I was unable able to move, unable to close my door. People walked in and out of my room whenever they wanted and injected me or examined my naked body. There seemed to be no regard for the fact I was a human. My private parts had become public property. My catheter was changed without anyone asking my permission – or without even a warning. But this. This was the worst intrusion of all. The only thing in life that I had control over was two half-hour television shows a day.

Two TV shows.

That was all I asked.

Melissa understood this, and respected that those two TV shows were *my* time and nothing was that urgent that it needed to interrupt them.

'How am I feeling?' I said, my voice becoming louder. 'I'm in the hospital. I've been here for nearly three months. I've been poked and prodded in every way possible and have had a string of operations that may not be over, so yes, I'm fucking brilliant! Now, hand me the remote, please.'

'So... do these operations worry you?' the woman asked.

'What do you want me to say?' I began yelling. 'These surgeries are fucking amazing, like going to a theme park. So exciting, like you never know what's going to happen! I love being cut open, I love being in pain. Fucking amazing – in fact, you should try it. Aren't you jealous you aren't in my position?'

Melissa was looking on in a kind of amusement mixed with worry, probably concerned that this woman was going to push me over the edge.

'So when you say you don't know what's going to happen, are you referring to death?' the woman asked. 'Are you worried about dying?'

Her question – her words – rocked me so deep to my core that I was speechless for what seemed like minutes. She was wrong about so much; I didn't know where to start.

What she didn't understand was that no child in a hospital bed is thinking about themselves all the time. It's not possible. Self-pity may be just around the corner, and even pure terror. But if you're in the fortunate position of having loved ones, and people caring for you, the last thing you do is focus more attention on yourself – or show how scared you are. *How can I sit here and say I'm scared when my parents are putting on a brave face for me?* The opposite happens, in fact. You become hyper-aware of the feelings and emotions of those around you. This is where I learned empathy, reading between the lines, picking up on the vibe around me, all the things that went unsaid. It's bad enough to be causing so much fear and pain, but the last thing you would want to do is to dwell on your own fears and misery and make anybody feel worse. You don't want people to worry more. You want them to worry less.

I was done. Done with this conversation and done with her. Conveniently my parents were not in sight, so I was free to completely lose it. Through a stream of tears I yelled, 'Who the fuck do you think you are coming in here? Get out of my room and give me the fucking TV remote!'

'But—'

'GET OUT! GET OUT! GET OUT!' I screamed. Melissa, who had disappeared momentarily, suddenly returned at the sound of my heart monitor, which was beginning to beep incessantly because my heart rate had spiked. My parents appeared just then, too, and quickly ushered the intrusive woman out of the room. Outside the door, I could see my dad having a word with her. My mum stood next to my bed and tried to calm me down, asking what had happened. But I didn't want to discuss it, and for the rest of the day it wasn't mentioned. I didn't know who the woman was, but I knew I never wanted to see her again.

The following day, my daily intake of pills seemed to grow. Mum examined the collection and commented on one of the pills. What was it? That's how we learned that the woman who had come to my room the day before was a psychiatrist. I had been diagnosed with depression – and the new pills were meant to treat this condition.

*Depressed?* Wasn't that a totally normal reaction to my situation? Thankfully my mum refused to make me take the antidepressant. As for me, I was outraged. At the same time, I did find myself questioning whether there could be any truth to it. *Perhaps this is what depression feels like? Is that why I'm so angry and upset?*

Very soon after, I was given much more to cope with. My infection had cleared and because of this, the doctors thought it was time to replace the shunt in my head. Another scan was performed.

But this time, upon looking at the scan, the doctors discovered something else: a brain tumour. It was the size of a strawberry.

We were told it had been there since my birth. I couldn't understand why they had never seen it, so, much like every other medical situation, they explained it with a childlike analogy.

'It's like you've been told that there is a treasure to find on the beach so you spend all your time walking up and down the beach, but have never thought to look in the sand. If you were to dig in the sand, you would have found the treasure sooner. But we didn't think to look in the sand because we didn't know the treasure existed.'

The good news: the tumour was benign. 'All they are going to do,' my mum explained, 'is remove it. But now we aren't sure whether you have hydrocephalus or not. Your symptoms could have been caused by just the tumour.

Or, you could have hydrocephalus *and* the tumour. After they remove it, they will find out.'

Surgery was scheduled immediately.

It was one of those times when it's impossible not to feel sorry for yourself – as if you've been singled out for torture. *Why me? Why me? Why me?*

My twelfth surgery in eleven years. Another surgery, another half of my head shaved, another scar. This was made worse when the surgery was suddenly cancelled, due to my low potassium levels, and rescheduled for two days later. Which meant two more days of worrying. If everybody thought I was depressed before, I was definitely depressed now. I spent most of my days sleeping, groggy under the influence of the multitude of drugs and withering away having not eaten actual food for the entirety of my hospitalization, surviving on the bare necessities of minerals being dripped into my veins.

My parents tried their best to keep my spirits up, and their own. My mum told me that the mistake made by the previous doctor – three months before – might have actually saved my life, as it had led to the doctors discovering this strawberry-sized tumour. Mum believed that everything happens for a reason, usually for a good reason. Silver linings were everywhere. But every time I was told that, I couldn't help but wonder if the reason was that I deserved it. Did I deserve this?

# 6

## Is perspective the solution?

I woke up after brain surgery in the same bed, same old corner of the ICU. I was parched – unspeakably thirsty – and couldn't move, or speak, or see much beyond blurry shapes around my bed without my glasses. After an effort to focus my eyes, I could see a vague individual-like shape sitting at the bottom of my bed, probably a nurse, which meant that it was night-time, because my parents weren't with me. I wriggled my hand slowly to find a button that would cause the bed to move and attract the nurse's attention, but my efforts were to no avail. A tube had been inserted down the back of my throat, stabbing with each swallow.

My entire head was wrapped in a thick layer of foam, presumably to prevent me from moving and causing damage to the stitches in the back of my head. They had shaved my head again. Could they not have warned me?

The pain was growing unbearable as the throbbing from the back of my head spread to the sides. I continued to stare at the figure on my bed, hoping that she would feel my intense gaze on her. As if I hadn't felt powerless enough, this was the moment I realized how truly incompetent I had become. I couldn't shower myself, couldn't use the toilet myself, couldn't brush my hair, move my body, speak or even see without another individual's assistance. As I lay there, I wondered how much time had passed. I waited for what seemed like hours, until the nurse finally looked up, and she spoke.

'Oh, you are awake? How are you feeling?'

I tried to say the words – and ask for water – but was unable. She must have known what I needed and explained that I was not allowed any water for the next two hours and that she could dab my tongue with a wet sponge. I mouthed whether ice chips were allowed, as I already knew the drill with this. Apparently enough time hadn't passed for ice chips. She dabbed my tongue and went back to her book shortly after, and I went back to lying there, wide awake until morning came.

Eventually my parents arrived. And over the coming weeks, the pain improved, as the wound in the back of my head began to recover, and I became more able. My abdominal muscles grew stronger and my days became filled with more events, and movement, as the nurses began preparing me to become mobile. I was supposed to be slowly attempting to sit up. Each day my parents and Melissa would help me to be in a more upright position.

They told me that it would relieve the bedsores that had been created from lying in the same position for months, but I still wasn't willing to try. I had no fight left in me.

This is when they turned to Angel, my furry friend. She was brought to me. Unlike all the previous times when she was put on my bed and lowered her head softly on my chest, instead, they placed her on my legs.

'We will have to raise your bed so that you can sit up and reach Angel.'

I refused. I knew what they were doing and it wasn't going to work.

'Every minute you stay lying down is a minute you're missing with Angel. Remember, you only have an hour with her.'

That was enough to spur me on to try. But as they went to the buttons to raise my bed, and my muscles started to engage with the raising of the bed, the pain kicked in. Having been unable to use my stomach muscles in months, it felt as if my stitches were being ripped open, as if a hand were tearing away at the skin and muscles. I screamed in agony as the bed slowly raised me. If it weren't for Angel I don't think I would have ever reached that point. The pain simply wouldn't have been worth it.

Slowly, I made small steps in the right direction. The following week I sat up off the back of the bed, the first time that I'd sat without my back supported in months. Then Angel was placed on the chair. It was only two steps away, and I had to be fully supported by two people either side. But sitting in a chair was a huge accomplishment, and my reward of playing with a dog was completely worth it.

Before I knew it, my recovery was in full swing, and I was learning how to walk again. Having to relearn this made me truly realize how much time had passed. I started slowly, with small steps around the ward, just enough exercise to challenge me. Every step hurt – and I would often feel weak after just a few paces. The only thing that kept me together was the support of all the others on the ward. It was overwhelming to be rooted for and encouraged by strangers, and to feel the warmth and excitement as I progressed. As I walked the corridors, they acted like I was in an Olympic race and in the lead. They cheered. They applauded. Soon I was walking alone with only the stand of IV drips to hold onto for support, and they did a Mexican wave as I hobbled past.

If you ever need motivation or inspiration, pay a visit to your local hospital or visit the children's ward of the ICU. I can assure you that the patients you will find there will be the most passionate and creative people ever. They have to be. A large number of them spend an unlimited number of days there and yet create ways to amuse themselves. I'd like to say they were inspirational in that they never complained, but that would be untrue – and unrealistic. What these kids had was perspective. Every day on rounds we were asked to describe our pain on a scale of one to ten, with ten being the worst pain. We all had our tens; those days when you thought it would never end and you started to forget what it was like to not be in pain. The days when all you wanted to do was scream 'why me?' and cry that everything was so unfair and you just wanted to be normal. But those days became increasingly rare the longer I was in the hospital.

Years later, I was asked to assign a number to rate a particular day in my life. I was on the way to a ski trip with friends, following exams at university. Our flight was cancelled and we were stuck at the airport for twelve hours and missed our connection. Right before we finally boarded our new rescheduled flight, a friend asked me, on a scale of one to ten, how I would rate the day, with ten being the best.

'Seven,' I replied. This caused great amusement among my friends, who were baffled by my judgement and how the extreme boredom and frustration of our day had resulted in such a high ranking. 'If this a seven, what the hell is your ten?' they cried out. But I had the benefit of experience, the benefit of months of agony, months of days that would be hard to rate at all.

Sometimes I still use the hospital scale to measure my day. And when I do, it doesn't take much for a day to feel utterly perfect.

# 7

## Why was I spared?

As the infection cleared, I was slowly eased back onto a full diet – after three months on a feeding tube or IV drip. Now it was time to eat like everybody else, by chewing and swallowing. Like a newborn, I started with liquids and proceeded to soft, bland food. Finally, the day came, the day I had been dreaming about: I could have my first real meal. Flavourful food hadn't passed my lips in months, and the thought of using my taste buds again excited me.

Without hesitation I knew what I wanted: McDonald's. It is no exaggeration to say that for months on liquid nutrients I had been dreaming of the McDonald's French fries, chicken nuggets and sweet-and-sour sauce. Ever since my godsister Julia had casually mentioned it on one of her visits to the hospital, I had thought of nothing else. Now, when I was told McDonald's wasn't a possibility,

I was offered a small slice of pizza instead. Good enough. I took what I could get.

One of the biggest perks of eating was that it would decrease the epic boredom of hospital existence. Eating gave me three more activities per day: breakfast, lunch and dinner. And as soon as the feeding tube was removed from my throat, it meant that I could brush my teeth – another thing that would take up more time. Savouring every second of these chores, I tried to expend as much time as possible on each of them – taking my time to order each meal, carefully imagining every item on the menu before eventually deciding, sometimes an hour later. With choices came more control. The ability to fill my day was a relief.

Less combative, I made friends with a hospital volunteer, a nice woman who had two dogs, grey and shiny schnauzers, which she brought around to visit with patients. One was named Rai Rai, the other Zee Zee. As I played with them, the woman told me about her job. She was a child psychologist, she told me, and her work entailed playing with kids and finding ways to determine how they were doing. She would sit with a young girl, for instance, and while they were playing with Barbie dolls, she would ask the young girl to tell her how the dolls were feeling. She said this gave her an indication of how the young girl was feeling too. With each visit, she told me more about her days – meeting with patients, playing, talking to them. Her methods, and her job, intrigued me. It had occurred to me that someday I might be able to have a job working with kids who were in the hospital. I could make them more comfortable by helping them to understand the procedures and the side-effects, whether it was a shaved head or scars.

When I mentioned this to the child psychologist, she explained what the word psychologist meant – and she shared with me how she had discovered her field and been trained. At that age, I wasn't entirely sure of the distinction between a psychiatrist and a psychologist but this woman seemed entirely different to the intrusive, impossible woman who had diagnosed me as depressed a month before. In my mind, psychiatrists were bad but psychology was the work of only the most compassionate and helpful people. With age, this belief would only grow stronger as I clung to this distinction. When people questioned me I would respond saying that psychiatrists only saw patients as charts and a list of conditions, whereas psychologists saw patients as complete humans with individual intricacies.

The conversation with that volunteer was the initial spark and spurred me on, giving me a new energy. I was going to be a psychologist when I grew up, and help children like me. Perhaps that was why I had gone through all of this – to be able to help others later. Recovery seemed closer, and I began to put more energy into it. I walked more, and tried to stay positive. I started to wonder: now that the brain tumour had been removed, was there a possibility of living without pain? Until that point, my migraines had always prevented me from fully taking part in activities – and in life. Was there a possibility that I wouldn't have hydrocephalus any more?

One morning, on the daily rounds, I asked the doctor this question.

'We have been wondering that,' the doctor replied, 'and the best way to find out is to test it. Since the tube is currently outside your body, we are going to clamp it off for a day and see how you respond. The good news is that if the experiment goes well, you won't need another operation.'

They began the experiment the next day. The tube that drained fluid from my brain was clamped and closed. Then, we just had to wait and see what would happen. My hope, of course, was that nothing would happen – meaning a future free of tubes and talk of brain fluid.

As the hours passed, I started feeling lightheaded. When I was unable to sit up, my daily walk was cancelled. A few hours later, a headache came on and the pain grew increasingly worse. When I asked for painkillers or morphine, I was told that this wasn't allowed. In order for the experiment to work, the doctors needed to know if my headache was going to continue. There was a chance that the pain was simply the result of my brain readjusting. In a few hours, they told me, I could begin to feel better.

I curled into a ball. My parents sat on either side of me and said nothing. For the last two weeks they had barely spoken to each other. I'd noticed small things: they would leave for lunch at different times, or only talk when passing things to one another. When they spoke to the nurses and doctors, they did so separately. I didn't ask why, but guessed that they had been fighting – probably about me.

'Why aren't you talking to each other?' I asked.

'Who says we aren't talking?' my mum said.

'We are talking,' my dad chimed in. 'Don't worry about us. We're fine. Just focus on getting through this.'

The situation had put stress on all of us, but mostly on them and their marriage. Never in a million years would they have admitted as much, though. While you're in the hospital, everyone tries to protect you from unnecessary stress or pain. Since my parents couldn't protect me from the physical pain, they tried in vain to protect me from everything else.

'There's nothing to get through,' I said. 'I just have to lie here and endure it. But it would be nice if my parents would talk to each other so that we could all have a conversation to distract me.'

The pressure in my head was becoming unbearable. I felt myself getting out of breath, and hyperventilating. A sudden pain in my chest made me gasp. The room began to spin and I lost focus. My eyes began rolling backwards into my head.

I heard Mum screaming. She ran from the room, calling for a nurse.

My dad reached for my hand. 'Stay with us. Stay with us,' he said to me. 'The nurse is coming.'

I tried to stay in the room, and keep my eyes looking forward and open. The nurse ran in and my mum exploded into full hysteria. The sound of her panic and emotional pain reminded me of when I'd seen the young boy die in the ICU a few months before. I was hearing those same sounds of grief and bewilderment; a raw, primal rage and fear.

Somehow, in that moment, I felt that if my mum could stop acting like that boy's mum, everything might be OK. Calming her down became my main concern. If Mum would calm down, I would live.

'Dad,' I said, 'just take care of Mum for me.'

I closed my eyes and suddenly felt relief, a great wave of calm – an almost hollow feeling – as if a pane of glass had appeared that separated me from the rest of the room. I could see everything and hear it all and tried to reach out to touch my parents but to no effect. But rather than being frustrating, I felt a sense of utter peace and an absence of time. This seemed to last for hours.

I would find out later that my heart had stopped. I had died. My mum's hysterical screaming had started when she saw the heart monitor flat-lining. She'd called for a doctor who had slapped and revived me, although I have no memory of that. Immediately, the clamp was removed from my tube. And I was alive.

At each new turning point in my life – when I got into university, when I kissed a boy for the first time, on graduation day, and every birthday that has passed since – I return to that experience. No one has been able to explain what actually happened. Or how I was able to know what was going on in the room even though my eyes were shut. But the feeling has stayed with me and pushes me forward. Why was I spared? *There must be a reason.*

The next day I had a new shunt put in. My thirteenth operation. I had always been superstitious about that number – because there are thirteen letters in my name, my first operation was when I was thirteen months old and, most of all, because I was born on Friday the thirteenth. Even though some of these were positive signs, the number scared me. These worries, though, remained silent worries. I feared that if I ever vocalized these worries, the words that would come out of my mouth would be considered my final goodbye. The only thing that consoled me was that I now knew that *the process of leaving this earth was peaceful*. But I wasn't ready to leave. Instead I hoped, wished and dreamed while I clutched Pogo with all my might. The banana-flavoured fumes filled my chest and sent me to sleep.

# 8

## Was I still lovable?

I woke up. First thought: I had survived. The curse of the number thirteen was over. Elated to have reached consciousness, even my thirst and the sharp unpleasant throbbing in my head was warmly welcomed. Before long, my recovery was in full throttle.

Impatience and agitation drove my rehabilitation; a sense of wanting to break free from the ICU and regain my independence. I was eager to leave the ICU, leave the hospital, leave Los Angeles, go home to Hong Kong, and eventually return to St Keyes and reconnect with classmates and friends. I felt this sense of urgency in every aspect of my life. On my daily walks around the ward, I often rushed, walking faster and faster, and feeling a strong wish to run, as if desperately trying to escape the boredom and isolation and sadness of hospital life.

By comparison, my days at St Keyes had seemed heavenly.

Since it was nearly the end of summer term, I found myself wishing I was back there, and daydreaming about all the celebrations that would be taking place. Exams would be over and the time of year that we had been told to look forward to would have commenced. Older girls often told us about this special post-summer exam period when the pace of studies would have slowed almost to a halt, replaced by sports days, fun projects and school pranks. Each year, the girls who were leaving would use these pranks as a way to say goodbye. One year, we were told that some girls rented an ice cream van to hand out free sweets on school grounds. Another time, school buildings were apparently sprayed with miles of Silly String and 'decorated' with loo roll. Events like these were looked forward to all year – and got the girls through their studies and exams. I longed to hear the school stories and be a part of it, even if I was half a world away.

Before texts and smartphones, if you couldn't access your email, connecting with classmates was almost impossible. There was only one computer in the ICU, and it was reserved for official use. On my walks around the ward, now that I was mobile, I stared at it longingly, watched the nurses doing searches and checking their mail, and saw that it was periodically left unused. I negotiated and bartered with Melissa to have just an hour to log on and check my email. She and I struck a deal: for one hour of computer time, I promised to walk an extra ten laps around the ward. When my hour arrived, I logged onto my email account and checked my inbox with great excitement.

It was empty.

Totally empty.

I returned to bed, unspeakably sad. Nobody had bothered to message me? Was I forgotten? I spent the rest of the day moping in my room, curled up in a ball, not talking to anyone until it reached 3 pm and the nurses told me it was time for my daily extra-long walk around the ward. The one I had promised. This was more than I could stand; I was too miserable to even consider it. School life had continued without me and this was a different feeling from anything I'd experienced before, when I'd spent Easter holidays in Hong Kong away from my friends. This was worse. Because I knew all my friends were together, having fun at the end of term. Not hearing from them, I felt friendless and alone.

The nurses refused to let me languish in bed. 'You must be getting tired of looking at the same four walls,' Melissa said. 'We thought it wouldn't be too bad if you walked around the whole floor instead.'

I knew this wasn't really allowed because of all my tubes and drains, but I didn't question why they were unplugging things, leaving only one remaining tube – my IV drip. So I went along, left the ICU and tried to enjoy the different views as I walked around other wards. The walls were a different colour. The nurses' stations were configured in different ways. But there wasn't much to be joyful about. Then, ten minutes into the walk, Melissa came up to me.

'Hey, they need you for another scan, urgently. Get in the wheelchair,' she said. I went along – too depressed to put up a fight. She wheeled me into the elevator and I noticed that she hadn't pushed the button for the floor where the scans and imaging areas were. Suddenly she was wheeling me in a new area of the hospital. Before I knew it, we were on the ground floor.

'Wait, where are we going?'

Melissa didn't respond. She didn't need to. In the distance I saw my parents. They were standing near to the entrance of the hospital. And just outside, beyond the doors, through the glass windows, I could see Julia, my godsister. She was standing with her dog, Frankie.

Over the last few months, Julia had been telling me stories about Frankie – and I had even tried to convince the nurses to let him visit me in the ward. But volunteer dogs had to have special immunizations. Frankie wasn't allowed inside.

'This is just mean,' I said to Melissa. 'You know I can't leave the hospital. Am I just meant to stare at him?'

'No,' she replied. 'We thought you might want to take Frankie for a walk.'

'Outside?' I leapt out of the wheelchair as fast I could, yanking my IV drip with me, and feeling a pulling sensation across my stitches.

'Easy now!' Melissa said. 'Sit back down. I'll wheel you out.'

It had been three months since I'd been outdoors. Three months since I'd been able to breathe fresh air or feel sunlight on my skin.

The electric doors of the hospital flew open. Melissa

wheeled me out, stopping on an island of grass. She lifted the footrests on the bottom of my wheelchair and I inched my way out of the chair, my feet slowly touching the ground.

I will never forget the feeling of that first touch of grass as it grazed the bottom of my toes. As I stood, the soft sponginess of the slightly damp earth felt like the simplest, yet purest of luxuries. The sun was shining on my back and I felt a soft breeze on my face. Hyper-aware of sounds, I heard birds chirping, the car horns and screeches from the street. I gripped my IV stand and pulled it alongside me as I hesitantly placed both feet on the ground, wobbling to find my balance. Julia handed me Frankie's leash and slowly, very slowly, I made my way across the grass.

Progress!

But after a dozen steps, I returned to my wheelchair for a break. Frankie was placed on my lap. As I stroked his fur, I noticed the skin on my wrist, around the IV drip tube, had a leathery appearance, as if it were shrivelling up and ageing before my eyes.

'You've been inside for so long,' Melissa explained, 'your skin is reacting to sunlight.'

It had been too long.


I was moved into a normal ward, where I shared a room with Nathalie, a fifteen-year-old girl who came for monthly surgeries to remove growths on her body – at least that's how she explained it to me. We spent evenings chatting and playing cards, one of my favourite pastimes that neither of my parents enjoyed. Our nurse, Matthew, was a gentle giant of a man with a California accent, like a character from an episode of the television show *The O.C.* He would occasionally join in our card games while Nathalie discussed her latest romantic adventures – how a boy had held her hand, or kissed her on the cheek. Matthew marvelled that we could find such innocent things so exciting, but at the ripe age of eleven, I devoured every word.

It wasn't just the romantic nature in me that was captivated. Hearing Nathalie's stories reassured me that someone could love you despite your illnesses, and most of all, despite your scars. There was still a small fragment of hope that my beauty hadn't been erased forever and I could still be lovable.

The freedom of the normal ward, and my increased mobility, meant that my antics and mini-rebellions were slightly more daring – and there appeared to be no curfew. Nathalie was my companion and accomplice. We would take turns wheeling each other and leaning the wheelchair back on the rear wheels as we raced down the corridors. One day, at two in the morning, midway through a game of cards with Matthew, we made a wager. If we lost, we would do our physiotherapy without complaining, but if we won, he would have to bring us a meal from McDonald's at the start of his next shift. And win we did.

There is no overstating what a big deal this was. After going for two months without eating any food whatsoever, over the previous month of my hospital stay I had been eased back onto a full diet very carefully – with liquids for a week, then gradually solid food. The most exciting thing I had been allowed to eat was chicken matzo soup from a nearby Jewish deli, which my mum had brought me. Now that I was finally able to eat whatever I wanted, my mind raced with fantasies. I wanted to explore everything I had missed in the last three months.

Most of all, what I really wanted was an In-N-Out burger – an LA delicacy that was talked about endlessly along the corridors of the ICU. But since there wasn't an In-N-Out close to UCLA, I settled on McDonald's yet again. Matthew assured us that as long as his shifts weren't changed, he would deliver on his promise. The next day couldn't come sooner. Nathalie and I woke up bright and early, awaiting Matthew's 7 am arrival, only to discover he had been moved off our ward and replaced with a stern elderly woman nurse, much to our dismay. No more dreams of McDonald's. With our new nurse enforcing the rules, this also meant no more late nights, card games or wild stories either. We were stuck in our beds to heal and rest, calmly and responsibly.

I found myself sneaking back to the ICU to visit Melissa or Rachel sometimes. It was hard to understand at the time, but somehow being away from the ICU made me sad. I missed the constant attention from Melissa and the hustle and bustle of the ward, even the sights and sounds and disruptions, the beeps of the monitors and other hospital equipment. My new ward was unsettlingly quiet – and boring. It was strange to share a small room with only one person, after spending the majority of three months in a large open space with a dozen other children. With the silence, I felt lonely and empty. Strangest of all, I had a growing jealousy of the people who were still back in the ICU. They were the important people, the critically ill, the VIPs of the floor, and while I was glad to be getting better, I experienced a strange wistfulness that I was no longer 'special'.

Melissa was happy to see me, and always briefed me on the news of the ICU. I learned that Baby Meg Ryan had actually gotten a new heart, which had excited her parents so much that they'd celebrated by buying pizza for the entire ward. But on the day that Baby Meg was finally ready to go home, the doctors discovered that her body was rejecting her new heart. It was such a cruel blow. Within a few hours, she was back in the ICU, and not long afterwards, she died.

That hit me hard. Here I was, getting stronger every day and preparing to leave, while the ICU was full of children who would never be better. Now that I was out, I considered all my complaints over the last few months in a different light. I felt a sudden pang of guilt realizing that what I had been through, in comparison, was nothing. I didn't have cancer, I didn't have burn scars that covered my face and body. I wasn't waiting for a new heart. And as far as I knew, I wouldn't have to return to hospital for future long-term stays, as Nathalie did. It was these constant reminders of the inequities of life that pulled me out of self-pity and drove me towards new resolutions.

My life needed to have purpose. I needed to feel that I had earned my good fortune. It was around this time that my decision to become a psychologist became more and more important to me – and brought me comfort. It wasn't just for Baby Meg. It was for all of the children I'd known or heard about who'd passed away during my stay in the ICU. For all the children I'd seen who were not going to get better, who were forced to live with chronic conditions and disorders or were waiting for new hearts or kidneys or lungs. Their little bodies lay for days on end in hospital beds, their skin unused to sunlight, their bare feet never getting to walk on the grass again. If only I could make a difference and improve their lives, and explain why I had been spared. I became determined: I was going to make my life count.

# 9
## Do we all need control?

Annabel was waiting for me in Hong Kong upon my return. I was tired from the long flight, and still not fully functional, but the chance to spend a week with my best friend from St Keyes was incentive to recover as fast as I could. She and I had planned this visit for months, long before I had become sick and left school. My parents had decided not to cancel it, hoping that Annabel would help ease me back into normality. She arrived in Hong Kong several days before I did, and spent time with my brother and Dad. When I got there, scabs from my head sutures were still falling out and it was still hard to walk for long, or quickly. On a trip to an amusement park, I sat on a bench below while Annabel enjoyed all the rides. I had very limited bursts of energy, but being with a friend fuelled me much more than expected.

We spent most of the time just catching up on all the

school gossip I had missed. Annabel told me about 'Muck-Up Day' when the oldest girls at St Keyes had gone to great lengths to pull off wild pranks. The last morning of the term, they had decided to bake something special for the whole school: delicious cupcakes. Upon arrival at breakfast, younger girls were surprised to find a tray of beautifully decorated cupcakes adorning each breakfast table. These were fought over and devoured. It was only discovered later, when it was much, much too late, that the cupcakes had been laced with strong laxatives. It was then that they found out what else the older girls had done: confiscated the loo rolls in all the bathrooms of the school buildings.

Also, there was a small patch of land in the middle of the school where a few horses grazed, owned by a nearby farmer. The graduating girls had decided to open the gate, allowing three horses to run free. They galloped down the hill in a panic as soon as the other girls in the school surrounded and tried to pet them. The 'leavers' had also filled the school courtyard with baked beans and hired a tractor to write a word in the grass of the lacrosse pitch: 'penis'. And lastly, hundreds of condoms had been inflated – enough to fill the chapel. This left Father Ted – the only teacher who used his first name, which as a consequence gave him an almost Madonna-like aura; no surname needed – totally distraught. He was an elderly and solemn man who led the daily prayers and considered the chapel his home. He had been found inconsolable after claiming the sanctity of the place had been ruined, leaving the teachers to clear the mess by popping each of the condom balloons by hand.

Hearing about all this mischief made me laugh, but as soon as I caught my breath, I felt sadder than ever. Annabel was only trying to entertain me, but the stories of St Keyes made me realize, acutely, how much I had missed. Before the age of Facebook and Twitter and other social media, three months away from school friends, particularly at the age of eleven, felt like an eternity. I did discover, happily, that girls had indeed written to me when I was in the hospital, but it had been so long since I'd used my email account that my inbox had been deleted. When my schoolmates didn't receive a response, they'd stopped writing.

Sensitive and caring, Annabel was quick to figure out that her stories about last term hadn't made me feel better, so she tried to lift my spirits by discussing in great detail what my return to school would be like – and encouraging me to imagine how the story of my three-month stay in a critical care unit of a California hospital would be received by our classmates. Before my abrupt departure, my popularity had been on the rise – caused, oddly enough, by my fragile health. This fuelled my hopes for a grand return, perhaps the biggest ever, and the possibility that I would ascend to a position of enormous status. I wanted this more than I can even say.

After Annabel left, the rest of the summer in Hong Kong went by in a haze. I recovered slowly and steadily. After a year of being away, I had no friends left in Hong Kong but I found solace in the company of my family. My brother and I spent hours playing Sims, a computer game in which the player creates a fictitious family, choosing their personalities and appearance, designing their home, and then totally controlling them.

Living in the alternate Sims universe was more enjoyable than living in the real world, as far as I could tell. I could choose what I looked like; my appearance was within my control. What did it say about my own newfound appearance that choosing to have scars in Sims wasn't even an option?

Between the four walls of my Sims home, I felt a kind of security that couldn't be attained in the real world. I was safe. Nothing bad could happen to me. Real life had so many risks – the risk of getting injured or hurt, the risk of having to return to the hospital. Rather than face risks, I immersed myself in the world of my own imagination, largely concerning St Keyes and the year ahead.

The decision to return to boarding school was never questioned or discussed. I'm not entirely sure why. My parents never broached the subject with me, or tried to encourage me to stay at home with them in Hong Kong. Years later, this became the subject of many teenage angst-filled arguments that I had with them. Was it smart to send me so far away after such an ordeal? Was I emotionally ready for these transitions? My parents confessed that while it might not have been the best parenting decision ever made, it felt too cruel to force me to stay home.

My dreams of returning to my friends, and school life, had seemed to empower me through my hospital stay. And after witnessing my close bond with Annabel, they believed that such friendships would inject some normality into my life after such a turbulent six months.

Their concern about my need for routine was only heightened when I began a habit of checking the doors repeatedly before going to bed. Although initially it seemed fairly benign, almost intelligent – showing a concern for safety – it was combined with a compulsive need to go to the toilet after each time I checked the doors. This obsessive behaviour was, as you can imagine, disruptive to my sleep. What my parents didn't know was that I spent most of the night lying awake and wondering whether I had unlocked the door instead of locking it, and fighting the urge to go back up to check again before contemplating whether I needed the toilet.

Eventually my parents noticed my nightly journeys back and forth from the front door to toilet to bed, then back again, and queried whether I needed to 'see someone', which meant a therapist. I went. It was only one session and a brief one. In the session, the therapist, a woman, explained that my need to check the doors revolved around a concern for safety. She theorized that this paranoia stemmed from the fact that I had a fear of seeing others in pain and this had manifested as a fear of being robbed which was due, in fact, to a fear of losing control.

As a remedy for the disruption to my sleep, she recommended I put empty Coke bottles behind both the front door and my bedroom door so that if anyone came in, the sound of the tumbling bottle would wake me up – and therefore I needn't worry. This rarely helped, as the carpet by the front door softened the noise and my deep-sleeping ability meant I never woke, even when my mother entered my room in the morning, followed by the commotion of Coke bottles being knocked over. What did bring comfort was the mere act of attempting to do something – seeing a professional who told me that I wasn't losing it after all, that my fears and paranoia were explained by stress and the ordeal I had just been through. Much to my mother's relief, the Coke bottles were eventually removed. From her perspective, putting them behind the doors was even more troubling than constantly checking the locks.

These obsessive behaviours never occurred if other people were sleeping in the room with me – another reason I looked forward to returning to school, where I would always have room-mates and, more importantly, where there were no locks that needed checking. I assumed the habit would hence fade away. And while the lock-checking did stop, my paranoia about intruders and robbers did not. Eventually I tackled it by not indulging the fears or behaviour. I told myself that I would outgrow it, so in the meantime I just ignored it – as a psychologist would say, I 'repressed' it. This meant that it would likely reappear at a later date, and it did.

This episode of heightened anxiety taught me several coping strategies that were guaranteed to put my mind at rest. One of these involved checking in on my parents before I went to bed. This would happen multiple times a night. If I knew my parents had fallen asleep, I would sneak into their room to check that they were still breathing, hovering at their doorway, initially hearing my dad snoring but having to pause a little longer to hear the quiet whisper of my mum's breath. At the time, this seemed perfectly normal. And if I could have outfitted both of them with heart monitors, like all my old room-mates in the ICU, I would have. Over time, like the door-lock checking compulsion, this behaviour lessened. Rather than having to continually check that my parents were still alive, I would only need to check once a night, just before drifting off to sleep myself.

Having spent the last few months with my body fighting itself, it only made sense that my mind wanted to join in too.

# SECTION TWO

# 10

## Do friendships stand the test of time?

Summer ended. It was finally time to return to England and my restlessness reached an all-time high. To distract myself from my worries, I decided to try to orchestrate a successful re-entry to school by transforming my terribly sad and painful experiences in the hospital into wild and exciting stories that would hypnotize and amuse my schoolmates – the gorier the better. I had watched Mum describe my surgeries to other people for years. She retold the stories with twists and turns, sensationalizing for effect and drama, and people were captivated by her every word. I assumed it would be easy for me to do the same, even though I had no practice at this. In fact, I had never really talked about my health or surgeries to anyone. I didn't know how hard it might be.

\*

Beginning the second year at St Keyes was exciting; a time when all the girls in my grade were assigned to a house where they would live for the next five years. I had gotten word that I would be living in Rodin, a house that was conveniently located in the main school building. Girls were sorted another way, as well. There were ninety girls in each year at St Keyes, and each of these were divided into three classes of thirty girls who would take lessons together for the duration of the year. I hoped against hope that Annabel was with me – and that I had been chosen for the highest level of maths.

There were still plenty of unknowns, but when I arrived in England with my mum, I was comforted by the familiarity of St Keyes. It wasn't the brand-new, unfamiliar place that I'd found a year before, when I'd started school. Now I was a seasoned pro and knew my way around, could navigate the names of the buildings, classrooms and teachers. Only occasionally did my mind drift to thoughts of Mrs Wright and wonder when our next encounter would take place. She had an elevated status at St Keyes, just a few positions below the headmistress, so I knew eventually I would see her, but with some luck, I hoped to have several weeks – if not months – without contact.

As my mum and I walked into Rodin House, I felt a growing sense of disappointment. Its design was misconfigured. Unlike most of the other houses, which were distinct buildings, Rodin was simply a collection of confusing rabbit-warren-type corridors at the top of the main school building. There was no front door, no entrance to Rodin House. The only indication that you had left the main school and entered a residence hall was a change of wall colour. When the corridor turned an unsightly, sickening shade of pink, you were in Rodin House.

Mum and I had arrived early that first day, allowing me a chance to explore my new room and get settled in. I remember how small I felt, how high the ceilings seemed, and how long and overwhelming the pink hallways and staircases of Rodin were. Venturing into my dorm, I learned that I was sharing rooms with only older girls – an intimidating discovery. When I looked at the door and saw four unfamiliar names, I tried to calm myself by thinking about how I would soon get to know them, as well as the other fifty girls in my house.

My new housemistress, Miss Naylor, appeared and introduced herself. An older woman with light-coloured, long hair that was clipped back in a twirl, she was poised and had a very similar stature to Mrs Wright, although with more elegance. She kindly invited my mum and me into her flat for a cup of tea. Adorning the pink walls were photos of her youth, capturing her beauty and a smile that had worn away with age. But I liked Miss Naylor. She seemed sympathetic – or at least I thought she tried to be.

Escorting me to my room, still empty, Miss Naylor invited me to choose any of the five beds for my own. I had been at the school long enough to know that that wasn't how it worked. The oldest girls always got preference and were first to choose which bed they wanted most. If I dare choose a bed out of turn, and it happened to be one that any of the other four girls wanted, I would be branded with a reputation for cockiness – the sort of thing that could follow you for the duration of your education, leading to a number of doors being slammed in your face, sideways stares and gossip.

With trepidation, I tried to guess which bed would be the least desirable. I looked for the customary drawbacks that younger girls had to endure – and asked for a bed that was neatly tucked behind the door, with slightly less cupboard space and a cramped bulletin board, reducing the number of pictures I could pin up. As I began to unpack with Mum, she expressed dismay about my choice of bed, but I reassured her that I liked my area small and cosy.

Mum and I finished unpacking and we said our goodbyes. Our goodbyes always made me feel uneasy, but as with all the other times before, I would soon forget once I was surrounded by my friends. I'd hoped this time would be the same. As soon as I closed the door behind her, I noticed how much pain I was in. I'd been feeling lightheaded all day – having climbed all those flights of stairs and walked those long stretches of corridors. I hadn't walked this far in months. I felt a headache coming on and tried to reassure myself that it had been caused by nothing more than exertion. To play it safe, I decided to lie down and rest on my bed.

On the other side of the wall, I could hear the bustle of

the girls catching up, laughing and giggling as they told stories of the summer. As an extrovert who didn't like being alone, I wanted to be sociable and outgoing – and join in the merriment. I enjoyed the constant hustle and bustle at school, with people always around to talk to. But my body was keeping me bed-bound, something that made me feel frustrated. But soon I was able to quiet my thoughts and drift off to sleep.

'Is everything OK?' I woke up to the voice of Mrs Corrigan, the house matron. It was her job to take care of the domestic affairs of Rodin. 'The girls in your dorm told me you were sleeping.'

'Yes, I'm just getting a bit of a headache,' I replied. 'I think I'm just tired.'

'OK, well – don't worry,' she said. 'I'll bring you up some dinner so you don't need to go downstairs.'

The school dining room was the social hub. All the other girls in my year would be there, catching up and laughing. While I really wanted to go down and say hi to my friends, and the other girls I hadn't seen in six months, I was pretty sure that taking dinner in my room, as Mrs Corrigan offered, was a wiser option. So I rested and ate quietly, and for the first time that I could remember, I felt lonely at the school. The previous year, my friends would have surrounded me and kept me company if I wasn't feeling well. We were a tight-knit group – and all the same age. Now I was rooming with girls who didn't know me. I was younger, an unknown, and probably annoying them because they had to keep their dorm light off as I was sleeping.

The following morning I rose slowly and dressed, hoping to find friends from my year in the main dining room and feel comforted. Looking around, I suddenly became aware of how many girls I didn't know. And the chatter! How did everyone have so much energy in the morning? I found my assigned table by the door, and greeted the other Rodin girls in my year. While I knew all of them, I had only ever spoken to two. Last year I had considered them friends, but I immediately sensed something had changed when they said hello. There was a hesitation and awkwardness, as if I were a stranger.

The conversation turned quickly to a discussion of which class we had been placed in, and which teachers we hoped to have. In just a few minutes these assignments would be pinned to the board, as breakfast came to an end. A single piece of paper would dictate the majority of our social life in the school year ahead.

Suddenly, a crowd formed in front of the board. The girls made noises, reacting to the news of their class assignments – mostly cheers. After making my way there, I was disappointed to discover that Annabel was not in my class – another bit of bad luck, since she wasn't in my house either. But I did see the names of a few girls whom I remembered and liked. I quickly headed to my form room, which was located near the courtyard of the main building.

As I approached, I heard the sounds of girls chatting and laughing, the room abuzz with cheerful conversations about holidays and summer trips. When I entered, the conversations stopped and the room fell silent.

All faces turned to me. I smiled awkwardly, turning to look behind me, confused as to what they were staring at. But soon enough I understood.

The bravest girl said it first: 'We thought you had died.'

# 11

## Who does revenge hurt more?

'Aren't you worried about seeing Mrs Wright?' one of the girls from my year had asked me that morning over breakfast.

In the six months since I'd left school, I hadn't heard from my old teacher. The only message she'd sent was directed solely to my parents. It didn't come after the discovery of my broken shunt, or my second surgery to implant the valve, or my third surgery to fix my intestines; Mrs Wright had only written my parents an email shortly after my diagnosis of a brain tumour. It was brief and offered an apology to them, telling them that she deserved to be given 'a slap on the wrist' upon my return.

The email from Mrs Wright took my parents by surprise. I had said nothing about how she had rolled me over like a corpse with her foot and dragged me across the classroom floor.

'What is she apologizing for?' my dad inquired. Not wanting to do anything that might interfere with my plans of returning to St Keyes, I told him that Mrs Wright had been a bit rude to me, that was all.

'She accused me of lying about having a headache,' I said. But privately, I fumed. What aggravated me most was that Mrs Wright had not written me a note or apologized to me, or expressed concern of any kind. She only cared what my parents might think. *A slap on the wrist, indeed.* I had more involved punishments and revenge scenarios playing out in my mind. She deserved a punch to the face, not a slap on the wrist. And one day, I told myself, I would deliver one.

Over breakfast that first morning at St Keyes, I was reminded that my scene with Mrs Wright had been witnessed by dozens of girls. Slowly, I began to hear their versions of it. One girl, who had been in a nearby classroom, recalled how Miss Naylor, my current housemistress, had stopped her lesson when the sound of my wailing startled her. This had sparked intrigue. Miss Naylor's entire class had begun peeking outside of the door to see what was happening.

'I can't believe she never apologized to you!'

'What will you do if you see her?'

Now, inside my form room, after encountering the stunned faces of my classmates – and being proclaimed 'risen from the dead' – I heard more impressions I had made at the school. Following my abrupt departure, the girls were told by our housemistress that I was returning to Hong

Kong to 'rest'. Each dorm had been asked to send a card to me, for all the girls to sign. Two months later, they heard I had a brain tumour. They had written emails, they said, but never heard back.

And since I was never spoken about by the teachers again, this led to a widespread belief that I was either dead or in a vegetative state. Another rumour surfaced and made its way around the school that I had had a brain haemorrhage, which led to me being renamed 'Brain Haemorrhage Girl'. It was assumed that I was never coming back. Next, all my belongings in my school locker and in my cupboard were sold off at an informal auction. Girls in my dorm had first dibs on my pens and notebooks. If they had lost their textbooks, mine were up for grabs. Or they would swap out mine with theirs, so at the end of the year, the textbook charge would be under my name, not theirs. My wardrobe was then ransacked and the rest of my possessions were gone as fast as I had been.

I laughed and took all this very light-heartedly at first. How silly the girls were! Can you imagine? *They thought I had died.* But when I left my classroom and had a chance to reflect, I realized how terrible this made me feel. Many girls had openly admitted to taking my things, and showed no sign of shame or guilt. It was funny to them.

Was that friendship by any definition? When they believed that I was dead or still haemorrhaging, they had swapped and bid for my clothes and school supplies – worn my clothes – and never given me another thought. Did the teachers forget too?

Meanwhile, the vague friendship group of my first year had disbanded. New cliques had formed – and were already tight. With the entry of new girls this year, the returning girls formed an alliance against them. I straddled an obscure boundary, since I was both a new return and an old girl. The result: I belonged nowhere. This was the hardest thing to accept, along with the feeling of being replaceable.

I also found it odd how uninterested the girls – and teachers for that matter – were in hearing my exciting and gory stories of survival. I had been totally wrong about that. Nobody even asked, 'What happened to you?' It wasn't until I said the words 'brain tumour' that I was able to generate even the smallest shred of interest.

This is how I learned the importance of having a brand-name illness. Tumours are tangible, imaginable things, an actual lump or growth in the body. But hydrocephalus is a complicated-sounding word, and a difficult condition to fathom. Despite the number of my surgeries, and the severity of the condition, very few people seemed to comprehend what it was – despite the fact that it's a common developmental disorder, as common as Down's Syndrome. Because I was still standing, looked normal, and didn't have c-a-n-c-e-r, people tried to change the subject as soon as the 'H' word was mentioned – presumably hoping to avoid an awkward moment when they would have to grope for the right sensitive words to say.

Nobody is born knowing what to say to a sick person. I understand that. And knowing what to say when you're twelve years old might be a rare talent. The only way I could potentially explain it was if a friend happened to see the odd episode of *Grey's Anatomy* or some other medical drama when it would crop up and I had the chance to say that it was what I had.

Except... once I was able to say *brain tumour*, the situation changed dramatically. Suddenly there was no awkwardness, scepticism or sense of disbelief. I wasn't a drama queen and exaggerator any longer. Mine became a story of triumph.

Now that the girls in my class realized that I was alive – and a brain tumour survivor – the next thing they wanted to talk about was our teacher assignments. *What if I had Mrs Wright?* We waited for our timetables to be given to us. We were *all* filled with dread, not just me. A kind of hysteria surrounded the fickleness of fate. Our teachers often dictated whether we were going to have a good year or not. But for me, the trepidation was tenfold.

As the timetables were slowly handed out, we studied them eagerly. There was a code of three letters that signified the identity of a teacher, usually their initials. When this code was deciphered, each girl yelled out the names of the teachers we'd have.

'Miss Matthews for English!'

'Yes!!'

'Mrs Simmons for physics!'

*'Nooooooo!'*

'Wait, who is ABM? Who teaches biology and begins with an M?'

Eventually my timetable reached me. As I quickly scanned it, I heard a voice from the back of the classroom call out: 'Michelle! We have Mrs Wright for PSHE!'

I looked down at my timetable.

There, under 'PSHE' were two letters: CW.

Catherine Wright.

Our first lesson was tomorrow.

My heart began beating faster in my chest. How *dare* the school give Mrs Wright to me again. She should have been sacked! But what infuriated me, created enormous entertainment for my classmates. With our PSHE class just a day away, they had a whole twenty-four hours to rile me up. Between each lesson, as we walked from classroom to classroom, or had breaks, the conversation revolved around this topic and stayed there, not budging.

There was a stream of questions:

'Will you scream or yell?'

'I thought you wanted to punch her and put her in her place!'

'Pretend to faint as soon as you see her!'

'I know,' another girl suggested, 'as she starts talking, walk out in the middle of class and see if she has the courage to come after you!'

'Kick her like she kicked you! Oh... *I would love to see the shock on her face!*'

'No! Egg her!'

The ideas became more and more dramatic as the day

wore on. While I took satisfaction in knowing that the girls were basically on my side, and I laughed along with them, a small tight ball of nerves sat heavily at the bottom of my stomach. With each passing minute, I felt more scared.

All those beautiful revenge fantasies whirled in my mind as I entered her classroom, but when I saw Mrs Wright's steely face, I froze.

'It's so nice having you back up on your feet, Michelle,' she said with a Cheshire-cat smile, exposing her yellow-stained teeth. It was a grin that showed cold calculation, not shame. Her eyes watched me very closely. Suddenly, I had a feeling that I had been put in her class deliberately, so she could keep me nearby, under a watchful gaze.

*So nice having you back on your feet.* I didn't know whether that was meant to be a joke or a pun, or even a serious remark, but in any case, it was in very poor taste. There were so many smart things I wanted to say in return. *No thanks to you.* Or, *I can't believe you still have a job.* Or, the most delightful one: *you won't be on your feet for much longer.* But the longer I waited to respond, the more I felt under pressure. I felt the eyes of my classmates on me – particularly the ones who had orchestrated that I enter the classroom last. They were waiting for something bold and vindictive.

Mrs Wright was motionless, standing with her cruel smile. How could she smile with such sharpness and ferocity? Suddenly I was flooded by a sense of humiliation and embarrassment, as if I had returned to being the little girl lying on the classroom floor. I muttered a few quiet words through clenched teeth, resorting to the tepid behaviour that St Keyes tried so hard to instil. The school was proud of its reputation for raising 'independent young ladies' but it had an archaic notion of what a lady should be: demure and docile, compliant yet successful. The aim was to be considered a prize possession until it was time to give birth – hence our curriculum came complete with cookery and textiles classes, to ensure that husbands could be guaranteed for all. The St Keyes way also meant voicing opinions only when they were acceptable and in line with the school views – not questioning the rules and regulations or disobeying figures of authority.

Was this all women were for? For a school that prided itself on instilling confidence in its students, it seemed that the message was more that our independence did, indeed, have a limit. Were we only allowed to express our independence when it was convenient?

At the age of twelve, it was hardly easy to confront an entirely corrupt culture and one so deeply ingrained. Due to Mrs Wright's status in the school, I wasn't able to express any of this overtly, nor my rage and feelings of injustice. Since returning, I had not even been asked how I was. Not by the girls, not by the staff. There had been frankly no interest in what had happened to me, nor any sort of apology or even signs of regret. The only acknowledgement of my absence was the fact that I had been removed from the top divisions of all subjects and placed in lower divisions – easier classes for less capable girls – a decision that felt more like a punishment. They justified it with the assumption that my intellect had decreased, despite the fact that post-brain surgery my IQ was re-tested to ensure no brain damage and I was actually found to have a *higher* IQ. Without asking, they had determined what I was capable of, and clearly Mrs Wright was going to be keeping an eye out to make sure I was sufficiently submissive.

And I suppose I was. But my anger surfaced in other places. Living at Rodin House with six other girls in my year group often gave rise to conflicts, due to our inability to escape each other's presence. The dorms changed every term so even though we weren't necessarily always put in the same dorm, we couldn't get away from the fact we shared the same house study and ate all our meals together. These were girls I wouldn't have chosen to spend my time with, and what made it harder was that the ones whom I would want to spend time with, like Annabel, were in different houses on the opposite end of the school. That, combined with the fact that we were also in different classes, made it even harder to bear the six girls being forced upon me.

Like sisters, we bickered and fought loudly. Most of my confrontations were with Carrie. She and I shared a number of friends and were always in competition. And because I was louder than anyone else, and probably had more to be angry about, with some frequency I found myself forced to sit in the office of my housemistress, Miss Naylor. My volume was 'unladylike'. My tendency to vocalize my feelings was deemed 'an ugly characteristic'.

'I understand you are an angry person,' Miss Naylor would say, her voice hardening to an accusatory tone, 'but that is not an acceptable way to speak to people. If you keep going this way, one day you are going to explode.' This was a common threat that she used with other girls, but it worked particularly well on me.

I would collapse in tears, apologize and say it wouldn't happen again. It was a pattern that I would go on to see in my adult life; I became aware that it was the norm to condemn women and shame them for their anger. As a female, anger was never an appropriate emotion, and I was taught to feel guilt around that anger. Guilt was digestible, more feminine, easier to control and manage, after all.

Slowly, I adapted to life at St Keyes, yelled less, and acquiesced more. Even though I wanted to stick up for myself, and to get even with Mrs Wright, I adopted a stance that would keep me out of trouble. When I exacted my revenge, it would be exactly the revenge I wanted.

# 12

## Did anyone care?

As the first weeks of term passed, there was still no acknowledgement of my health or hospitalization. It was as if my stay in the hospital had just been a bad dream. My fantasies over the summer in Hong Kong with Annabel of regaling St Keyes with my surgery stories had vanished after the first week back. Walking into each new class, with each new teacher, my expectation of sympathy had begun to reduce.

As for my friends, I had lost them – to other girls, other friendship groups. They hadn't just forgotten about me; it was worse than that. They didn't care. After the first few weeks, I stopped expecting any of them to ask how I was. Only my piano teacher seemed happy to see me.

Mr Bernard was one of the few male members of staff; a tall, attractive Frenchman with a brilliant sense of humour. He was as passionate about his pupils as he was about his music. The year before, although I had been playing the piano since the age of five, I had arrived at the school with a mysteriously low ability. Mr Bernard found it impossible to believe that I had toiled for six years at the keys and gotten almost nowhere. I had trouble completing even Grade One piano pieces, which launched Mr Bernard on a personal crusade to see me achieve much more, because he believed me capable of greater accomplishments.

I had looked forward to resuming my private lessons and continuing our bond. Funny, energetic and occasionally flamboyant, Mr Bernard's company would, I knew, be restorative and reassuring. He kept me interested in music, and kept me laughing. In between his motivational outbursts, we had often discussed non-related subjects from television shows we liked, like *The X Factor*, to the latest gossip in the staffroom.

'Michelle!' he exclaimed, bursting into the practice room, pronouncing my name in a fully French way, like in the Beatles song that I liked so much. 'What happened to you?' he asked. 'One day you were here, and then you weren't! All they said was that you were ill and had left the school.'

He rattled off his experience of confusion and concern at warp speed. I paused to recover from the shock of finally being asked how I was, and then began explaining what had happened – first this operation, then that procedure, another operation, scan after scan, all those months in the ICU, then the discovery of the brain tumour...

It produced the reaction I had hoped for: shock,

sadness, surprise and sympathy. Mr Bernard was warm, caring and wholly human. Being with him reminded me of all the things that were otherwise absent at the school. After spending weeks being treated as if I were invisible, I had started believing that maybe what had happened to me wasn't such a big deal after all.

'*Mon Dieu*! I'm so sorry, Michelle.'

Walking out of my piano lesson, my mind was swirling with questions. Why was Mr Bernard so freely emotional and caring, yet the other staff so strangely silent? It was gratifying, and moving, but the words of sympathy weren't coming out of the mouth of the teacher who owed me an apology. I tried to put the pieces of the puzzle together – to solve the mystery of my homecoming to St Keyes. It felt like a punishment, as if I had done something wrong. Mr Bernard's reaction was the normal human response; but even nice teachers at the school seemed muzzled and mute.

Then I realized the difference: Mr Bernard was not a staff member of St Keyes. He was just a piano teacher who was brought in to give private lessons. He was not privy to school politics. He behaved in accordance with his own rules of conduct. Later, Mr Bernard told me more details about how Mrs Wright had discussed my illness in closed-door staff meetings, and I developed another theory: perhaps the headmistress and school board had been concerned about a lawsuit and charges of negligence. If so, Mr Bernard would not be aware of this.

*

My next lesson that day was English – the one I dreaded most. To make things worse, my teacher was Miss Naylor, my housemistress. I worried about the impression she must've been assembling of me while teaching my worst subject. It was only a matter of time before she would conclude that I was dense.

Our lesson that day was moved to the computer room, which usually signified an upcoming project. The girls in my class whispered with curiosity when Miss Naylor entered and announced that we were going to write our autobiographies. She explained that this would be our largest assignment to date and would require us to write a minimum of ten typed pages, create a title, design a front cover, write a short description or blurb, and bind all the printed pages so that they formed a proper book. Everyone was excited by the prospect of this, finding it far more fun and exciting than the classic works of literature that we were ordinarily assigned, such as *Pride and Prejudice* and *Macbeth*.

As some of the girls began to type away, giggling as they wrote, others discussed what title they would give their book. My mind was totally blank. Looking at the computer screen, I had no idea where to begin. After the bell rang and all the girls flooded out of the computer room, I approached Miss Naylor. 'I'm really struggling,' I confessed. 'I don't know where to begin…'

In all honesty, I was too embarrassed to admit that I didn't understand my own life – or exactly what all of my surgeries had been about. I hoped that she would have some advice for me, a bit of inspiration or motivation – things that teachers are supposed to be good at.

'Just give it your best shot,' she said quickly and began packing up her files. She rushed off with a quick, 'I've got to go,' followed by, 'Don't be late for your next lesson.'

As the week wore on, the assignment weighed more and more heavily on me. In hopes of getting under way, I began work on the front cover of the book in art class. I had chosen my title, 'Thirteen', but having never been the artistic type, a design wasn't coming to me easily.

'Argh, I wish I knew what to do,' I said aloud, to anyone and no one.

'You should do this,' a girl next to me said with a laugh. Then she drew a stick figure lying down, with crosses for eyes and a tongue sticking out.

'What? I look dead.'

'Exactly!' she giggled wickedly, getting me to laugh along with her. We doodled together as I drew the number thirteen.

'Why thirteen?' she asked.

'Because I was born on Friday the thirteenth, I have thirteen letters in my name, my first operation was when I was thirteen months old and I've had thirteen operations.'

She fell silent, as our drawing continued. 'Wouldn't it be funny if you died in 2013?' she said. 'Then your life would almost be circular.' I laughed along with her, but later wished I hadn't.

That evening, I called my parents with all my questions. What had my first seven operations been for? I remember a vague mention about a surgery on my eyes – was this true? What exactly did the tube in my neck do?

Their answers involved hours of explanation, after which I had learned an overwhelming amount. And with this new knowledge, I began writing my story.

> Before writing my autobiography, I had not fully under-stood my life. It was all a blur. I knew I'd had thirteen operations but I didn't really know why. I knew that I had a tube but I didn't really know where. Most people understand their life, but mine is very hard to explain – especially to a seven-year-old…
>
> But now I understood. I understood ALL the facts. The pieces had fallen into place.

The autobiography – a total of fifty pages and 10,000 words, roughly five times longer than the stories my class-mates were turning in – was merely a collection of facts. The story of my life could not have been more flat. In all those hours of writing, it had never occurred to me to describe how I felt.

Immediately I began a revision, thinking that I would drop in some emotion where I could. Starting from the beginning, I got to the first event in my life that should've triggered emotion – falling ill and fainting for the first time. I asked myself: *how did I feel?* I couldn't think of an answer. I flipped forward in the story, to the moment where I died and was revived in the hospital – a moment that should have triggered a wave of emotion. But instead,

I felt nothing. It was alarming that even in my attempt to remember those emotions, I was unable to. All I experienced was complete detachment, almost as if it hadn't been me who had experienced them. Almost as if I had taken in everyone's reactions to my experiences and now had this desensitized reaction myself.

But I knew, in order to get the grade I wanted – A* – that the story needed emotional content. Miss Naylor had said as much. So I began inserting sentences that conveyed feelings, here and there.

When I got to the story about my heart monitor flat-lining, and dying in my hospital bed, I added the sentence: 'I was scared.'

And the discovery that I had a brain tumour was accompanied by the revelation that 'I was sad'.

When I encountered the hospital psychologist, I inserted: 'I was angry.'

These were the reactions that I knew I should've had. That's all. If I had ever truly felt that way, I couldn't remember it now. It was almost as if the surgeries had happened to one person – me – and the feelings had happened to somebody else. It would be many years before I would realize that this disconnection from feelings, or from the memory of feelings, was very common – in fact, it was expected – for anyone who had been through a traumatic or life-threatening situation. It was part of *survival mode*. Denial is a survival mechanism, and it can cause a continuous sense of doubt about what has actually occurred. Many events can feel as if they were simply imagined.

Survivor's guilt is another common expression of trauma; a sense that you don't deserve to be alive, where you question the good fortune to have survived a situation that many others didn't. Another survival mechanism is hyper-vigilance – in my case, all the door checking, lock checking and concerns about security. At the time, though, none of this seemed like abnormal behaviour. Even my lack of emotion didn't raise alarm bells in my own head. It just seemed a little odd. But as is the case with survival mode, I didn't dwell on thoughts like this for long. The key is to keep moving forward.

Believing I had described enough emotion to satisfy Miss Naylor, I turned my book in – feeling certain, because I had put so much time into it, and written more pages than anyone else, that I'd get the grade I wanted. The following week as we filed into English class, I also expected to be praised for my bravery in sharing the intricate details of my gory adventure. Sitting in class, I watched Miss Naylor as she passed back our books and I waited for her praise, or an acknowledgement of some kind. Then my book came back with a Post-it note stuck on the top. Miss Naylor had written: 'B+. Good effort, love the positive and optimistic approach.'

Those words stung. 'Positive' and 'optimistic' wasn't what I had been aiming for. At other schools, getting a B+ may have been considered good, but at St Keyes anything less than an A★ came with disappointment. I had witnessed many girls cry over such a grade. I wasn't going to cry. Instead, I became enraged. After class, I returned to

Rodin and crashed through the door of the study with a complaint already coming out of my mouth. 'Miss Naylor is such a bitch!' I cried. 'She gave me a B+ when I wrote 10,000 fucking words!'

'Ha-ha, you have Naylor for English,' one of my house-mates called out. 'Can't imagine having to stare at her face three times a week.'

'No wonder she's a housemistress,' another girl said. 'Can you imagine how miserable your life must be to want that job? To actually choose to be here?'

There were times when the brutal culture at the school – the blatant disregard for the humanity of our teachers and house-mistresses, or anybody else for that matter – comforted me. When you have feelings to bury, and keep buried, there's no better place on Earth. I tucked my autobiography away in a pile of papers, and eventually it found its way to the bottom of a trunk, then into a box, then somehow onto my bookshelf. Many years passed before I read it again and could see, so plainly now, that the positivity and optimism, so glaring and bouncing, were false and jarring. The word 'luckily' had been written at least once per page, as I described how mistakes that the doctors had made had been fortunate accidents, and how each hospital stay led towards the discovery of my brain tumour – as though it were a golden egg or the ultimate prize on a scavenger hunt.

# 13

## Am I fat?

Eventually I had to join in PE lessons. It was the season for lacrosse, the sport I hated most in the world. Balls flying at head-height were scary enough, but a lacrosse ball could do serious damage – as demonstrated when one of my friends had wound up with a black eye. I couldn't understand the appeal of playing such a dangerous game that seemed to me to be an arena for taking out personal grudges. I had barely built up the courage to leave the house over the summer in Hong Kong, much less the strength to enter the mosh pit of the lacrosse field. Adding to my reluctance, I dreaded the inevitable social humiliation of being unable to keep up with the game – and being seen so publicly running behind my teammates, gasping and out of breath. Even getting across the school grounds in time for lessons was difficult enough. The surgeries and months of hospital confinement had taken their toll.

The whole day before that first PE lesson, my mind spiralled with worst-case scenarios – flying lacrosse balls, headbutting – and the fear of ending up back in hospital. Before I knew it, in a moment of mild hysteria, I told my PE teacher that my doctors in the US would not allow me to play contact sports for six months, as I was still 'recovering'. When my parents were asked to provide a note confirming this, they went along – which surprised me – and I was removed from playing sports. This was a great relief. Since the school had showed so little ability to look after my wellbeing, it seemed like a fair compensation to lie and manipulate the lacrosse situation to my advantage.

At the first ever PE lesson, which I attended, the teacher warned the girls that lacrosse practice went ahead whether it was raining, hailing or snowing. This made me feel even better about not playing. I assumed that I would be allowed to skip the entire lesson and return to study at Rodin. But something else transpired: I was informed that I would be sitting on the sidelines, and then, after the matches were over, walking around to collect stray lacrosse balls. It was a grave disappointment, but one I could live with.

As I sat on the sidelines, I was the subject of envy and occasional praise. Other girls, who hated lacrosse as much I did, passed me with whispered taunts and sighs of approval. Occasionally, I was joined on the sidelines by other girls who had gotten 'off-games' notes from their matrons, and when they learned that my note kept me from playing for the next six months, they expressed even more profound envy.

But one girl, Eleanor, had a rather unexpected reaction. 'Aren't you worried about getting fat?'

'You're just jealous,' I retorted.

Eleanor was an effortlessly beautiful girl – stunning – and it surprised me that she would be so focused on my appearance. I'd understand if it was someone like me saying it, but did even beautiful girls think about their appearance? My weight had never been something I thought too much about. Growing up, there had been comments about it, like I was described as having 'baby fat' a few times, but that was to be expected when you grew up in Hong Kong where everyone was considered fat no matter how skinny you were. When I lost weight in the hospital, people remarked that I looked 'weak' and 'frail' – and told me to eat more. Most people, like me, remember these kinds of comments, and file them away in the place where we are forming opinions about ourselves and how we 'should' look.

*Aren't you worried about getting fat?* Later, Eleanor's remark returned to my mind, like a mantra. Sitting on the sidelines during PE lessons did exactly what she predicted: my weight began to climb.

When I had entered the hospital, I weighed 52 kg – or 115 lbs. When I came out, I was 42 kg – or approximately 90 lbs. But in less than three months after leaving the hospital, doing nothing but playing Sims at home in Hong Kong, and now sitting on the sidelines of PE, I weighed 72 kg – almost 160 lbs. A total gain of 30 kg – or nearly 70 lbs – in a very short time. The explanation wasn't just my inactivity. It was due to the effects of being fed from a tube for so long, which had sent my metabolism into starvation mode. My body had been reset to retain all extra calories. The consequences were terrible. My clothes didn't fit. My naturally lean body no longer looked like my own, and panting while walking up stairs became my new normal.

Worried about what was happening, after two months on the sidelines I told my housemistress that I was feeling more capable and strong and wanted to be able to play sports again. To convince her, I revised my original lie and said that the six months that the doctors required me to refrain from physical activity were meant to include the three months of the summer holidays – meaning my return to PE was only around the corner.

It was true that I hated lacrosse, but alongside the threat of gaining weight, I also resented sitting on the sidelines. It reminded me of my hospital experience and made me frustrated that yet again, I was being kept away from my peers – this time out of my own doing. This feeling only worsened when our PE lessons involved netball: my favourite sport. I asked my neurosurgeon to write a note allowing me to play netball specifically. But after all my lies, which had apparently been so convincing, the teachers decided it was too big a risk. When the netball season started, with each game that I watched, rather than played in, the irony of the situation hit me. All those months in the hospital, when I was stir-crazy and so desperate to leave, my greatest fear had been becoming paralysed and having to sit on the sidelines of life.

And yet now my fear of landing back in hospital from the impact of a lacrosse ball was instead what had paralysed me. My concocted lie now felt more like a straitjacket. My housemates in Rodin came to regard me as a weepy fragile flower, often stating that I took things too seriously. I was quicker painted as a girl who was sick and over-sensitive and needed special treatment. I was determined to rectify that.

My first PE lesson back as a full participant was cross-country running, which coincided with the most unpleasant winter weather conditions, from pouring rain to snow. Even worse, each girl's ability was ranked. The previous year, I had suffered humiliation when I finished towards the end of my class, so this year I was determined to improve. I was motivated – more than any of my classmates – and this drive overshadowed the dread I felt about running and being ranked again.

I knew I couldn't compete with the best girls, but I was determined to at least beat my previous time from the year before.

Standing ready at the starting line, I saw the long stretch of greenery ahead of me, lined with trees – and in the distance, a steep climb. The whistle blew and we were off. Alongside all of my friends, I felt pure joy at being able to use my legs for the first time in what seemed like ages. A cold breeze touched my face and I felt a surge of energy. As expected, the fastest girls began to pull away from the pack. Mud splattered as the herd of girls clambered forward, squelching through it, everyone attempting to maintain momentum.

My breathing grew painful, despite the energy in my legs. I came to a halt and more girls passed me. Facing some steep terrain, I began walking. Climbing through the forest, I found it hard to look up, and difficult to catch my breath.

When I emerged from the forest, I was relieved to be on flat land again. I looked up. No one was around me. No one was even in front of me. I was alone.

Even though my jog had already slowed to a walk, I remained adamant, refusing to give up. Quitting was not an option and had never happened during a cross-country lesson. The last thing I wanted was to go down in school history for that. I stopped intermittently to catch my breath. My lungs felt tight and sore. It had been a while since I had seen anyone but I kept moving forward, tears streaming down my cheeks. I thought about the humiliating scene ahead – my arrival at the finish line, dead last.

Then, suddenly, I saw another person ahead of me, not too far away. But wait. It was a man. And he was running towards me. A teacher.

He approached me, jogging, and explained in a breathy voice that they were worried that I had gotten lost. He encouraged me to keep going, and reassured me that he would keep me company. I didn't have the energy or breath to explain that his company only added to my embarrassment. Finishing last was bad enough, but being chaperoned by a member of the staff was so much worse.

At twenty-nine minutes, I crossed the finish line, twelve minutes behind the next-to-last girl. On the sidelines, I could hear whispers and complaints about being kept waiting, and how hungry everybody was for lunch. Even when people congratulated me, it oozed pity. Never had a teacher had to go back and find someone, let alone run alongside them to support them in the completion. The phrase 'I want to go bury myself in a hole' came to mind. If I wasn't the 'fat friend' before, I certainly fit the stereotype now.

Yet there was more embarrassment to come.

This came with gymnastics. For my entire life, anything that required being upside down, sideways or flipping over quickly had been problematic, due to my shunt or tube. I couldn't ride on rollercoasters or hang off the side of my bed – never mind cartwheels, handstands and mid-air flips.

In the first year of gymnastics, the lessons had involved more dance-based movements, so I had been able to participate. But in my second year at St Keyes we had advanced to vaults, trampolines and headstands. I expected that I would be asked to sit and observe on the sidelines, once again, but instead – like my lacrosse experience – I was given my own special assignment to do in the corner of the gym: sausage rolls, and if I was feeling extremely energetic, something called a 'teddy bear roll'.

Sausage rolls involve lying on the floor with your arms and legs outstretched, then rolling up and down like a log of play-dough. Teddy bear rolls were done while lying on your side, in a crunched, seated position, while holding your legs. In other words, you look like a loser. And my classmates were not about to let me forget it.

But there was another aspect of PE that I had grown to hate even more.

Changing rooms.

# 14

## Do you have to stare?

Once upon a time, when I was little, a changing room in any shop was a place of joy, where new clothes arrived as if by magic, brought into the small space by my mum or a shop assistant. I would try on these new clothes, pulling them off my body if they felt too clingy or scratchy, and barely look at myself in the mirror. When I was really young, what mattered was how the fabric felt on my skin or how a certain colour attracted my eye.

Under the harsh overhead lights in a shop changing room, nobody looks their best. But as a little girl, I looked at myself only long enough to get the gist of a new outfit. It was just a quick glance. But that innocence and lack of self-consciousness evaporated eventually. And I remember exactly when it did.

When I was ten, I had been invited to a birthday party for a school friend. The invitations were handed around the class, and the envelope contained a blue card – I can still picture it – describing a pool party: my favourite. As the date approached, I decided that I wanted a new bathing suit. Many of my friends had abandoned their one-piece suits for a new trend. Their little bodies were beginning to develop and rather than hide this, I guess they wanted to show off their new maturity. Not wanting to be left behind, I had asked Mum if I could have a bikini too.

Mum didn't answer me right away. She seemed to be avoiding this conversation. I had no idea why. I continued to dwell on my need for a bikini, though, and finally she relented. At a store in our local shopping mall, we found the section dedicated to summer: flip-flops, sarongs and every kind of swimsuit. I was beside myself with excitement. As we perused the swimsuit section, I found a white bikini with fluorescent pink and orange glittery stripes. My heart skipped a beat. I couldn't wait to put it on. I raced to the changing room, in anticipation of how beautiful it was going to be.

I looked in the mirror, feeling very proud and beautiful. Then I spun around and danced out of the changing room to show Mum.

'Look! It's incredible!'

A fake smile was plastered on Mum's face. I couldn't help but notice how uncomfortable she looked. Confused, I turned and noticed two people standing to my side – a woman and her daughter. They were frozen in place, just staring at me. The mother held a hand over her mouth to conceal her shocked expression and intake of air. But I heard the gasp. A look of sadness and pity crossed her face. I followed her gaze to the middle of my stomach. She was looking directly at my scars, the network of crossing lines that formed a chequerboard on my belly.

A sudden sense of shame began to overwhelm me, almost drown me. I ran back inside the small changing room, determined not to cry in front of these strangers or my mum. But trying to contain such a strong emotion only transformed my embarrassment into rage. As soon as I was alone in the dressing room, I decided that – no matter what – I would wear the white bikini with the fluorescent pink and orange glittery stripes at the birthday party. And nobody was going to convince me otherwise.

Surprised that I still wanted to buy the bathing suit, Mum gently urged me against it. 'Michelle, let's find a pretty new one-piece for you to wear.' But her attempts were futile. My mind was made up.

The next day, I arrived late to the birthday party. Rather than joining the other girls immediately by the swimming pool, I whisked into the changing rooms in the clubhouse of the birthday girl's apartment building, and proceeded to get into my new bikini. I walked out to the pool without any sort of cover up, not even a towel. As soon as I appeared, the faces of my girlfriends changed. Their eyes darted away – and a silence fell on the pool area. I hadn't realized, until that moment, that none of them really knew anything about my surgeries. Perhaps they knew that I was often ill and had to miss school, but certainly not the details. Especially not the surgeries. I had never mentioned them. There had been no reason to.

I greeted the birthday girl, who was wearing that same tight smile that I'd seen on my mum's face the day before, in the shopping mall. The girl was frozen, as if stunned, as if she were witnessing a car crash or something else equally horrific. A sick fascination appeared to have taken hold of her. Then, when she came to her senses, her face melted into sadness and pity, an expression that began spreading through the group like a virus. Very soon, their pity enveloped me. And I could hear the whispering of other girls who didn't know me – they were curious and asking questions. Suddenly it felt as if the entertainment for the party had started. And I was it.

I ran back into the changing room and started crying. I wished I could just peel the scars off like a plaster, or wake up and discover they were gone. A sharp feeling of hatred for my body came over me. It was strong and raw. It was an I-could-stab-you-with-a-pitchfork kind of hatred. But I wasn't going to let anybody know that. Upon the announcement of lunch being served, I quickly wrapped myself in a towel and pretended nothing was wrong. Everyone else did the same. As soon as lunch was over, I called Mum and told her I wasn't feeling well and wanted to go home.

After that day, there was no turning back. My insecurities and scar-consciousness grew – along with an urge to change myself. On a trip with my mum to the pharmacy, I found a jar of 'scar-reducing' cream and secretly purchased it before she could see, charging it to our family's account and tucking it into the waistband of my jeans. I began applying the cream repeatedly throughout the day, and again before bed. With each trip to the pharmacy, I found more creams and scar remedies – including a purple one whose colour vanished when rubbed in, which seemed like proof it was working. In a matter of weeks, I had quite a collection, and every chance I got, I dug into my cupboard of mystery lotions and gels and began applying them. A few months later, my mum discovered my hidden jars and bottles and calmly explained that they would not erase or reduce my scarring.

Not wanting to give up hope, I searched online for more options, stumbling across the mention of 'plastic surgery'. I broached the subject with my parents, but they grew quiet and thoughtfully explained that, at ten years old, I was much too young for that. My body was still growing. But they said that if I still wanted it when I was sixteen, it would be an option. They also warned me that the procedure would require another hospital stay.

'Do you remember your last operation, three years ago?' my dad explained.

I nodded, unsure how this was related.

'Well, the recovery process would be the same. You'll be in a lot of pain.'

My desire for plastic surgery was suspended, but it gave me some solace to think there were options for later on, when I was older. It made it easier to accept my scars if I thought of them as temporary. Just six more years and they could be made to disappear...

Now I had more scars than ever – seven cuts across my stomach, all parallel and neatly done, the four on my head with two matching ones across my ankles from an intern performing a blood test gone wrong. But the biggest incision, created during the emergency surgery in California, had created a deep fold at the bottom of my abdomen that protruded from my otherwise lean frame like a bizarre roll of fat. I was haunted by this roll. Looking fat was seen as such a sin – especially in such a vanity-obsessed school. The worst part was that it was even noticeable under a T-shirt. And up near my collarbones, I had two new scars from when the tubes had to remain outside of my body for the three months in hospital. They were relatively small but, because of their location, they were visible with scoop-neck tops. More often than not, I forgot all about them. That changed one day, as I dressed in shorts and a polo top for PE.

'Ewwww, Michelle, cover your nipple! That's so gross!'

I looked down at my polo top and saw nothing. I looked at the girl making the sounds of disgust.

'What are you talking about?' I asked.

'That thing there,' she said, pointing in the direction of one of the small scars near my collarbone. It was a lumpy scar, so I suppose the confusion was understandable. By now, though, an audience had formed around us. At the mere utterance of 'nipple', the girls around me started laughing.

'That's not a nipple,' I said. 'It's a scar from one of my surgeries.'

The changing room fell dead quiet. One of my friends broke the silence, reminding us it was time to go to class. And the girl who had declared I was showing my nipple departed as quickly as she could, avoiding eye contact with me for the rest of the day. My scars weren't only ugly and disturbing; they couldn't even be discussed without shame and embarrassment – mine and everybody else's.

During another PE changing-room session, I was standing in my underwear and talking to a friend when I turned to see a younger girl staring at my stomach, so absorbed with my scars that she hadn't noticed I was staring back at her.

'Do you want to take a picture or something?' I snapped.

Taken by surprise, she picked up her tennis racket and fled, mumbling apologies on the way out. The changing room exploded in mixed reactions. Some of the girls in my year – particularly the more popular ones who liked to pick on the younger girls – found it hilarious and were laughing. More sensitive girls felt that I had been too harsh, reminding me that a stern remark from an older girl can be felt deeply by a younger girl. It's true, I could have been kinder. But in that moment, while various discussions were under way, I had only one thought in my mind: *will I have to deal with this my entire life?*

# 15

## Is this friendship?

Annabel was in Crow Hill, the farthest house away from Rodin, at the top of a very steep slope and a fifteen-minute walk for me. It had a reputation for being home to sporty, popular girls. Because of this physical distance, and not being in class together, my time with Annabel had been reduced to a quick hug in the corridor on our way to lessons and the occasional lunch when our breaks happened to coincide.

Since Rodin was my home – and would be for the next five years, until my last year of secondary school – I spent most of my time with the girls there. I knew Maisie the best, but even so, not that well. A quiet girl with big green eyes, soft frizzy brown hair and a rosy complexion, Maisie and I had shared a dorm the previous year, our beds directly next to each other, but we hadn't spoken to each other much.

The other Rodin girls in my year were definitely not shy.

We were all strong, ambitious characters who struggled with enhanced levels of competitiveness and frequently butted heads. Most of us were talented in some respect – either academically or musically or athletically – and everybody had an opinion. Due to my various dramas in PE, and being perceived as crying wolf about my headaches whenever it was convenient, I became regarded as hypersensitive and the girls began to tread lightly around me. Rather than argue with me, or tease me, the girls usually tried to not engage – or they ended our conversations with a sigh.

Everybody except Carrie, that is. A tall, brainy girl who looked down on everybody – both literally and figuratively – Carrie had a distinct need to compete with me and everybody else. She gloated about her victories and good grades. She enjoyed making others feel inferior. In the Rodin study room, while the other girls laughed and gossiped, she was always buried in the corner studying, perfecting her assignments and only surfacing for mealtimes or to borrow someone's homework. Meanwhile, she would never offer to help other girls with their studies. She was afraid they might get a better grade.

At lunch one day, as we took our places at the assigned table and began digging into our food (in that indelicate fashion found in all boarding schools, where meals are scoffed down as quickly as possible in order to get back to work), one by one we noticed that Carrie was sitting in an awkward position. She had written '100' on the back of her hand in orange highlighter and was holding her fist so it was visible to us.

'What's on your hand, Carrie?' a girl called Esme asked, casually.

Esme was the resident free spirit, easygoing and comically disorganized. She could barely keep track of her books long enough to even attempt to study, much less be irritated by Carrie's perfectionism.

'You mean *this*?' Carrie smiled, as if surprised anyone had noticed. 'Oh, it's just the mark I got in my history test. I got a hundred per cent, that's all.'

We all fell silent, trying not to give Carrie the attention she so desperately craved. But I wasn't able to stay quiet for long. I knew a few people at the table weren't happy with their history test marks and Carrie's bragging and insensitivity were hard to take. But just as I was about to speak, I felt a strong kick under the table.

Stephanie, sitting next to me, silently mouthed the words 'shut up'.

No more than thirty minutes later, when lunch was over and I was deep into my homework in the study room, Esme appeared from around the corner. She sat down on top of my desk and glared at me.

'What the hell are you doing?' I asked.

Esme lifted up her hand. On the back, she had written '101' in orange highlighter. 'Guess who I am?' she said. We erupted into laughter and before we knew it, everyone in the study room was walking around with '101' on their hands.

As we gathered around our table for dinner that night and began to eat, we posed on our arms in the same awkward manner that Carrie had done at lunch.

'Why does everyone have a hundred and one written on their hands?' she asked. Her flat tone, and total lack of comprehension, only made it funnier.

'Oh,' Esme chimed in. 'It's just what I got in my maths test.'

'But you can't get a hundred and one per cent!' Carrie replied, rising to the bait. '*Who gave you a hundred and one per cent? That's ridiculous!*' As her frustration began to build, we all started to snigger, eventually crumbling into hysterics – until someone revealed that we were just pulling her leg.

'Well it's not funny!' she cried out, then picked up her tray and left in a huff.

Eventually the other girls learned to leave Carrie alone or ignore her. But I couldn't. This led to constant squabbles and other confrontations and we became enemies. Time after time, the girls of Rodin told me to 'let Carrie be Carrie', but I was never able to follow that advice. Sometimes just the sight of her could drive me over the edge.

The acrimony, teasing and competitiveness in Rodin wore me down sometimes. We knew each other's weaknesses all too well, and this hadn't led to a sense of affection, much less trust. It was a long five years until I found a friend group I really loved – and who loved me back. There were times when I dreamed of changing schools – and openly talked about it. Surely there must be a place where true friendship existed, rather than open cruelty? But I was afraid of what an unfamiliar school might bring. And there were always reasons to stay. I was optimistic,

I guess, that my situation would improve. I told myself if I stayed another year, I would become a 'housemother' at Rodin. And if I stayed one more year after that, I could look forward to the privilege of being the head of dorm, where I would be left in charge. Then, if I kept going at St Keyes, I would leave Rodin for the last year of sixth form, when all the girls in my year would have our own single rooms in different dormitories. Sixth form meant much more independence. And you could run things at the school, be a leader, and have a title like 'prefect' or 'officer'. That was *real* power. Deep down, I knew I wanted that.

# 16

## Can you just stop eating?

As I went through the stages of puberty like any other teenage girl, my physical appearance started to bother me. I became more aware, more self-conscious. I had steadily gained weight in the three years following my operations while the girls around me had become thinner and thinner. The school environment – probably not unlike any other boarding school full of stressed-out, type-A, ambitious girls – was a breeding ground for bulimia and anorexia. At Rodin, it became an epidemic.

It started innocently. Several girls had decided to try a crash diet the previous year, when we were thirteen. They would go to great lengths to avoid food, signing in for attendance at every meal but not eating anything, sometimes skipping lunch and dinner completely. It became a game. They used tactics like pushing food around the plate so their dieting would go unnoticed. I'm sure quite a few of them were also purging when they did eat anything. There was even a toilet that was coined the 'bulimic toilet' at Rodin – one that had a proper door on it, so girls could vomit in peace.

As their weight loss became more dramatic, the girls worried about how to keep it from being detected by the school nurses. Every term there were health tests, 'Heights and Weights' – simple weigh-ins, done by the school, to ensure eating disorders were not missed. The night before their check-up, girls chugged down bottles and bottles of water. The next morning, they wore the heaviest clothes they owned. Some resorted to adding ankle and wrist weights to their skinny frames and disguising them with oversized tracksuit bottoms and hoodies. These tactics often worked – and the matrons somehow didn't seem to notice the faint aroma of bile that lingered around the bulimic girls, like a noxious cloud.

Mealtimes became frustrating for me. When the dinner bell rang it took forever to find anyone to sit at the table with me and actually eat. On the odd occasion that all the girls would come along to the dining room, the conversation revolved around weight loss and calories, the girls expressing enormous pride about how well they were doing on their crash diets. They felt great about themselves – now that their ribs were showing and their collarbones protruding. It was hard not to sit there and sigh with boredom.

Eventually, though, I started to succumb. After a year in this super-thin hothouse, it was almost impossible not to focus on my own weight. Before going into the hospital, it had never been an issue or struggle. But now, my clothes felt tighter which only accentuated the stomach roll created by my biggest scar. After weeks of quietly analysing myself in the mirror, in the house study one night I finally went public with my frustration. 'Urghhhh, my stomach is so gross!' I cried out. 'I think I need to go on a diet.'

'It's simple,' Stephanie chimed in from behind her desk. 'Just stop eating.'

'You mean like you did last year?' I asked.

'Yup, just like that,' she replied. 'Look, we can do it together, just for a weekend. It'll be really fun. You have to dodge the teachers and not get caught. Also, I haven't done it in a while, so I could do with losing a few.'

'Maisie, you in?' Stephanie called out.

Maisie agreed. Before I knew it, I had entered into the game. The hunger games – literally.

We began that weekend. The bell rang for breakfast and took me by surprise. I wasn't sure what I was going to do – or how to avoid eating. When I arrived in the dining room, Maisie and Stephanie were already there. They were carrying full plates of bread and bowls of cereal.

They demonstrated their technique and I watched the theatrical performance. Maisie got up with a slice of bread to put in the toaster. Stephanie filled her cereal bowl with milk. Maisie returned with her toast and started spreading it with jam. Stephanie clanged her spoon around her bowl, lifted it up a few times, as though eating, but never placing the spoon in her mouth. It was mesmerizing. Their acting was so subtle and elaborately thought-out. How easy it was, while everybody else was chatting and chewing, to go unnoticed.

Stephanie stared at me, and then raised her eyebrows to give me the signal. It was time for me to partake in the charade. I walked slowly to get a boiled egg and took my time purposely forgetting cutlery, resulting in an extra few walks back and forth to pass the time. I cut my boiled egg open, peeled the shell, walked over to the toaster, hovering over it then burning it so I could spend time scraping the ash off before slowly spreading butter on my toast, then ripped it into two pieces. Before I knew it, the bell had rung. First meal (not) done!

Throughout the rest of the morning, as my hunger became distracting and uncomfortable, I found comfort in a sense of accomplishment. With no musical or sporting abilities, and just a few academic ones, this warm feeling of pride was nice – and it almost made my stomach feel full. Best of all, I was playing a secret game with my friends. Fuelled by a newfound sense of camaraderie, and my own enthusiasm for pushing my body to new extremes, by the time twelve hours had passed, no food had entered my mouth.

The next day was slightly harder, but my friends praised and encouraged me. I liked the attention and had only one bite to eat at lunch and one bite at dinner. When I went to bed hungry, I felt proud. The gurgling of my stomach was almost comforting. Stephanie and Maisie encouraged me to stay on track, while their diets became more lax.

They had lost all the weight they wanted to lose in just a few days, but said they were going to continue to support me until I reached my goal of shedding twenty pounds in a month. When we were all offered a chocolate bar after our netball match, they caved, but I kept going – and felt strong, secure and confident. The weekend flew by and I hadn't eaten a thing! Before I knew it, the weight was coming off.

The only problem was the mood swings. When I didn't eat, I became lethargic and irritable. When I did eat, even a forkful or two, I experienced a sugar rush. Suddenly I was too full of energy – and would return to the study room at Rodin and run around, silly and hyper. Carrie found this especially annoying, being the studious type who took her schoolwork very seriously. One day, post-lunch, she blew up. 'For fuck's sake,' she yelled out, 'just because you've eaten for once in your life, we don't all need to know about it!'

I pretended not to know what she was talking about. But she continued. 'I'm going to tell Miss Naylor that you're missing meals. You're so bloody annoying when you do eat, but when you don't, you're even worse!'

Would she dare tell Miss Naylor? This was a pretty large threat. There was a rumour going around that if another Rodin girl was diagnosed bulimic or anorexic, Miss Naylor would lose her job. By this point, a number of girls in the house had been hospitalized for eating disorders. Several of them had even left school and been put into that most esteemed rehab facility, The Priory. It wasn't just

Rodin, either. Having an eating disorder had become such a common thing at St Keyes that if you noticed someone was missing in class, and a friend revealed a departure for The Priory had taken place, there was little to no reaction – as if we believed we might all eventually end up there.

At the same time, none of us had any idea about these conditions or how they started – and how dangerous our game really was. There weren't clinics or classes to educate us. The focus at St Keyes was forward drive – towards academic and athletic excellence and achievements. We felt we were always competing for first prize. A number of the girls had high expectations placed on them by their parents and this only escalated as the term came to an end. GCSEs approached. The special St Keyes cocktail of competitiveness and need for attention, combined with high-pressure parents and a cruel school culture, created the ideal place for eating disorders to fester.

That day in the study room, I pointed out to Carrie that I was only eating like the majority of the girls at school, and our argument continued to escalate until she stormed out. 'You're an arsehole,' she called out as she left. 'You always were an arsehole and you always will be!'

But that wasn't the end of it. Later that evening, when she asked if I was coming to dinner with the rest of house, I felt pressured to go – and eat. This gave Carrie satisfaction, and after that, she began checking to see if I was actually eating or just moving food around on my plate. So I ate, not wanting to prove her right. Regardless of whether she meant well or was just trying to score another victory over me, my starvation diet had ended. I guess I have her to thank. I've often wondered if I would've gone down a slippery slope towards anorexia without her intervention.

God knows, the teachers at St Keyes weren't paying attention. At 'Heights and Weights', when it was recorded that I'd lost twenty pounds in the space of a month, no alarms bells appeared to go off – and nobody came to sit me down for a talk. Clearly, they weren't concerned since I didn't look anorexic. But the following month, as Carrie hounded me to eat and keep eating, and I gained it all back – plus an additional ten pounds – it was an entirely different matter. Alarm bells sounded. One evening, when Miss Naylor saw me pulling on the waistband of a skirt because it had become too tight, she told me to come to her office the following day. Her amateur psychoanalysing sessions were notorious; she would meet with girls one-on-one and make them cry.

'I've been concerned about your weight,' she began as soon as I arrived. 'I've noticed it piling on slowly, and combined with the yelling I've overheard, I can tell you must be a very unhappy person.'

In our past one-on-ones, which usually involved arguments that I was having with the other Rodin girls, I'd tried to stay dry-eyed, but to no avail. The longest I'd ever gone without crying in Miss Naylor's office was two minutes. But now that we were discussing my weight, almost instantaneously, a tear escaped from my eye.

'You have so much anger inside of you,' she continued. 'It's going to eat you up and one day you're going to explode. We can't do much about that, but at the very least we can address this weight issue. To be honest, I'm very proud of you for not being anorexic. Any other girl would have resorted to starving themselves by now.'

*Was this supposed to be a compliment?* She seemed to be sorry that I hadn't developed an eating disorder and gotten skinny like the other girls at St Keyes. It seemed ironic that just a month before I had done that precise thing but because I hadn't attained the result of having a dangerously low BMI, my symptoms hadn't appeared problematic.

Miss Naylor continued her spiel, describing my weight as 'getting out of hand'. Tears rolled down my cheeks as I was made to feel terrible about being a size twelve, and a perfectly normal weight for a fifteen-year-old girl. No wonder so many girls wound up in The Priory.

Desperately wanting to 'help' me, Miss Naylor offered a diet plan. She discussed foods to avoid, how the caloric system worked, and why I needed to eat healthy snacks and keep nuts and seeds in my room. She suggested that I begin this diet under her watchful eye, which turned out to involve random checks, when she would pull out the weighing scale to study my progress. Scales weren't allowed in our school, with the exception of the ones within the medical centre for 'Heights and Weights'. This was due to the prevalence of eating disorders, but this, Miss Naylor believed, would be an exception.

The constant monitoring of my weight made me more obsessive about food than ever. Another downside of Miss Naylor's diet plan was that she suddenly felt entitled to make public comments about my eating habits at any time. At dinner, she criticized me for eating a potato. At breakfast, she would notice the bacon I had on my plate. Midday, she discovered a cookie in my hand and there was an outburst. The school provided these cookies, a speciality of the kitchen, at our 10 am break – an irresistibly chewy concoction of sugar and chocolate. Other girls grabbed as many as they could; I took only one and savoured every crumb.

'Michelle, what's that you're eating? A cookie? Hand that over now!' Miss Naylor shrieked.

Embarrassed, I handed over my cookie. And as soon as she left, the girls around me burst into hysterics.

'Sucks to be you.'

'I have three cookies, you have none.'

'Give me that!' I yelled, snatching one from the girl's hand.

About a month into my stint as her dieting guinea pig, I had cookery class where we all baked a chocolate cake. Afterwards, I was carrying it very proudly back to Rodin, walking to the house kitchen, when I passed Miss Naylor in the corridor. As soon as she saw me, she called out, loudly: *'Michelle, stop eating!'*

I'd had no intention of eating the cake. I was donating it to the house for communal consumption, and had already promised slices to friends, who were waiting in the kitchen. 'Oh, I just came from cooking class,' I began to explain.

'Michelle, stop eating!' she interrupted.

'But it's not for me, it's for—'

*'MICHELLE, STOP EATING!'*

An entire kitchen of girls heard her shrieking. After that, it was mimicked over and over – a running joke for years – at mealtimes, or whenever food was near me. It was repeated so frequently that one afternoon in the common room, when Esme was strumming on her guitar, she began singing, 'Michelle, stop eating!' A Facebook page was even created with the same name: 'MICHELLE STOP EATING'.

I laughed along, seeing how ludicrous it was. And for a time I felt comforted by the humour. But it was still a joke about my weight, my size… my body.

Eventually Miss Naylor got tired of having a pet project that wasn't successful. She let me know that unless I started 'taking this seriously' – by which she meant her diet plan – she would give up on me. Her snarky comments began dying down, along with her monitoring every single item on my plate. I was extremely, extremely relieved. I didn't need her interference. I didn't want her help and definitely hadn't asked for it. I wanted to dine in peace. My supposed 'weight problem' was just that: mine.

# 17

## Are all boys like this?

Soon, all the food and friendship dramas were replaced by another obsession: boys. By Year 11, the girls in my year were actively discussing who had kissed a boy (quite a few), who had a boyfriend (fewer), and there were extremely long and involved conversations about the one girl in our year who had actually had sex. We all knew these details by heart.

As with everything else, boys became a competition – even though experiences with them were extremely limited, since most of us had spent our school years sequestered in an all-girls environment. Hoping to socialize us properly, the school began organizing occasional 'socials' for girls as soon as we were twelve – but not too many so as not to distract us from our studies. A boys' boarding school would come to St Keyes – or vice versa – and we would have dinner together, followed by dancing. Other more 'adventurous' ideas were employed to prompt us to inter- act with our young male visitors – gimmicks and games that were considered a warm-up exercise to eating or dancing together. One of these alternative suggestions was a 'quiz' supervised by Mrs Wright.

Since returning to school after my hospitalizations, it seemed only fitting that she was present for my first encounters with boys. For the first social, all the girls in my year boarded a bus that took us to a boys' school far away. To kick off this presumably miserable event, while the bus rumbled along the country roads, Mrs Wright stood in the aisle and imparted her wisdom:

'Now, the boys you will be meeting might not be the most "slightly" of sorts,' she announced in her stiff but carefully modulated voice. 'They most probably will have acne. And they most certainly will be smaller and shorter than you. But my, will they blossom into fine young chaps one day and you will do yourself a great service to befriend them young. These spotty, short boys will sprout into strapping men whom you could one day go out with – and perhaps even marry.'

As the social unfolded, her predictions about the boys proved true. And there was very little actual socializing to speak of. A clear divide had been created in the middle of the dancefloor with all the girls and boys separated. This encouraged the boys to be as disgusting as possible. They stood close to the clear partition and, as if we were zoo animals they were trying to shock, made faces at us, burped and picked their noses. It was a horror show none of us would ever forget.

For the next two years I avoided the sign-up sheet for socials, not wanting a repeat of the previous social. I couldn't understand why anyone would want to endure that kind of evening again, yet nearly all the girls did. Unlike me, they held on to the hope that Mrs Wright had discussed about these boys flourishing into strapping young men, but I was less than convinced. The choosing of which girls would attend was done via a lottery to keep the numbers down. I stood back and watched our entire year – all ninety girls – race to add their names to the sheet and scream with joy when they were chosen to attend. They began planning their outfits immediately, and as the date drew near they would run around Rodin trying different things on, making a final decision and seeing Miss Naylor for approval. (After which, tops were lowered and skirts were hiked up.) Hair and nails were prepped, followed by careful deliberations about makeup. The girls who weren't chosen to attend looked on jealously, awaiting their turn at this new form of competition.

All except me. By the time I was fifteen, the competition for the most kisses, dances, dates, or any other contact with boys – especially sex – brought only dread. One kind of social did tempt me, though. And I tried it.

'Speed dating' was just as it sounds – a series of rapid one-on-ones when a girl and a boy sat across from each other and had three minutes to meet and talk, before a bell rang and the boys moved on, kind of like musical chairs. The idea had intrigued me, and seemed more fun than the traditional dinner and dance. And since this social was located at St Keyes, it didn't involve an endless bus ride and I knew I'd feel more comfortable.

Unfortunately, as it turned out, speed dating only cemented my impressions of the opposite sex. Every single male I met in these three-minute bursts was rude, arrogant and childish. As soon as they plonked themselves down in a chair opposite me, something offensive would come out of their mouths.

'So,' one boy began, in a deliberately bored voice. 'I guess you're from Hong Kong?'

'Yes, I am,' I replied. Since every single Chinese girl at St Keyes was from Hong Kong, it didn't seem like that clever a guess.

'So you know my grandfather,' he said with supreme arrogance.

I gave him a blank look. It amazed me how many boys wanted to investigate social credentials and play the name game.

'He owns the biggest casino in Macau and is from one of the richest families,' the boy went on, 'so you must know him.'

I raised an eyebrow, then slowly swivelled to the side to look at Maisie, who was deep in a conversation with her boy of the speed-dating moment.

'Green or red apples?' the boy was asking her.

'Green.'

They'd been firing these strange questions at each other for the last minute, giggling at their responses, until she noticed me looking at her.

'What are you doing?' she whispered, leaning into me. 'Turn back, Michelle. You're being rude. I'm talking to my guy – you talk to yours.' Then she resumed her game of choices.

'Chocolate or popcorn?'

I rolled my eyes and swivelled back to look at my three-minute date. Was I really meant to continue this silly game?

The night only got worse from there. When we moved on to the dinner portion of the evening, the girls were told to take a seat at a table, and the boys would shortly follow. The girls took their places, keeping empty chairs between them, where the boys were meant to sit. Entering the room, each boy stopped to study the tables, finding the most attractive and popular girls and then fighting with each other to sit with them. I watched as forty boys attempted to cram into two tables, pulling chairs away from eight other tables of girls, until the teachers had to intervene. You'd think that was a positive development, but it wasn't. Instead of politely making conversation, the boys spent the entire night yelling back to their friends at other tables and ignoring most of the girls near them.

The real games began as soon as the dancing portion of the evening got under way. The silent goal among the St Keyes girls was to see how many boys you could 'pull' in one night. This involved the most graphic kind of make-out session, with tongues not restricted to inside the mouth. Lips didn't just meet lips; the boy's mouth surrounded the entirety of a girl's lower face – potentially her chin as well. And in order for a kissing session to count, it had to be done in the most public way possible – even if girls had to clamber to the top of the tiered seats along the wall with a boy so that their kissing was sure to be in clear view of the other girls and teachers.

The teachers circled the room like security guards, ensuring they monitored the toilets as well, to make sure that no 'funny business' was going on. But the older girls made it their mission to escape to darker and more secret locations – and their stories and rumours, like having sex in the chapel, made them overnight stars of their year, and eventually the school, once word got out.

Kissing a boy in a public way brought a status hike. But the ultimate victory went to any girl who managed to snag an actual boyfriend at one of these events. Most girls didn't, but the pressure was so tremendous that they lied about it – telling embellished or entirely fabricated stories of encounters with boys and new 'boyfriends' in such detail that they seemed almost believable. One girl kept us all enrapt with a story about how her handbag had been knocked over at the airport and a charming boy with one green and one blue eye appeared to help her. As he bent down to collect her handbag, he discovered that tampons had spilled from it and were all over the floor. In the most gentlemanly way, he handed them back to her. Later, he wound up being on her flight – and she discovered that he had put his phone number in her phone. Each week there was a new, equally delicious instalment.

She wasn't alone. Other clever, imaginative manoeuvres were employed. Several St Keyes girls created entirely fake Facebook accounts for their nonexistent boyfriends, whose faces were Photoshopped onto celebrity bodies. Sometimes forged love notes were shared. A girl once claimed that a boy had sung a romantic song to her and sent her a recording of it in an audio file. But she had sung it herself and electronically manipulated the recording to make it sound two octaves lower, and like a male voice. These creative measures were inevitably suspected to be lies, but rarely acknowledged as such. To extract herself from this web of fiction, the lying girl would usually make up a romantic story of separation or tragic break-up, which was often more intriguing than the original lie.

I couldn't understand why a girl would want to fabricate a fake boyfriend, much less date a real one. I had no interest in adding another field where I had to compete to be on top, especially when I knew that with my body, and my scars, I was already in a losing battle. It seemed easier to be apathetic than confront my very real fear of being rejected. I continued to try everything under the sun to avoid the socials – and it drove a wedge between me and the other Rodin girls. Their interests were turning to house parties in London, now that we were allowed longer leaves from the school at weekends, increasing the opportunity to meet boys. With ceaseless fascination, they spent all day and night analysing various potential boy-friends. I got tired of hearing the boys' names – and the 'cute' nicknames the girls had given them.

'Michelle, leave the room,' Stephanie said to me one night when all the Rodin girls had come back from a social. 'We're going to talk about boys and you just wouldn't understand. You see, unlike you, we are actually growing up.'

I remained silent for once, not knowing how to respond. I had been growing sick of this superiority, which was based simply on the fact that they had an interest in boys and I didn't. I stared at her emotionlessly, my face demonstrating how unimpressed I was with her being more experienced than me. Oblivious, she continued in a patronizing tone: 'Socials are for three things – the three B's. Boobs, booze and boys.'

'Boobs?'

Carrie chimed in: 'Yeah, that's what socials are for, duh. Showing off your body.'

I'd had enough. Just as I turned to leave the room, closing the door behind me, I heard Maisie say, 'I told you she couldn't handle it. She's embarrassed at any mention of boys.'

She was right about that. Over the last year and all the talk about sexual conquests, I had grown more and more uncomfortable, assuming no boy would ever find me attractive. The thought of a boy someday seeing my scars filled me with terror and Carrie had just confirmed that all a girl was good for was her body. What did I have to offer, then? While I told myself that my scars were souvenirs of bravery and courage, and a reminder that I felt grateful just to be alive, I couldn't help but hate how deformed the scars made my stomach look – as if I had three rolls of belly fat. The other girls counted calories and discussed bikini waxes and manicures, but I was left with an unfixable problem.

Avoiding socials and silly house parties was easy enough. But what would happen when I went to university? I wouldn't allow myself to even think about it.

In Asia, it's acceptable to comment on a person's physical appearance openly. Instead of saying hello, it's customary to begin conversations with sentences like, 'Wow you've got fat!' So trips home to Hong Kong always brought out my insecurities. Over the holidays at home, each family friend made mention of my larger size and it stung. Size twelve in petite and skinny Asia was considered obese.

One day, while sunbathing with a group of my mother's friends on the front deck of a boat, I decided not to remove my bathing suit top, as they had. I wanted to keep my scars covered up and avoid unnecessary attention.

'Take your top off!' my mother's friend Samantha called out to me. 'No need to be shy!' Not wanting to turn my scars into an even bigger deal than necessary, I obliged, removing my top slowly. I was relieved to see that all the women had their eyes shut and were chatting, paying no attention to me. I resumed my position, and then I noticed

Samantha turning towards me, eyes wide open and holding her cigarette up to get my attention.

'You know, Michelle,' she started in, 'you are so gorgeous. You have the most beautiful eyes and your lips are stunning.'

I was very flattered, and beamed as I thanked her. But she wasn't finished. 'If only you would lose some weight. Boys really don't like girls your size.'

This left me speechless. Couldn't Samantha see my body? *It was covered in scars.* It seemed incredible that she would go on about my weight, when other things were clearly a bigger problem. The irony was highlighted as she went on describing the health consequences of my weight, while smoking cigarette after cigarette. Yet her first comment was what stuck with me. If I could somehow get boys to like me and my scars, would I start to like them too?

Not long after returning to St Keyes for the first year of sixth form, I was going to lunch with a few of my friends after our PE lesson. We were just about to walk out of the sports centre when Tatiana, a beautiful girl with distinguished features, caught her reflection in the glass door.

'Fuck, I'm so fat,' she said sadly. 'Look at how ugly I am.'

My first instinct was to comfort her, as I normally would, and say something like, 'No way! Look at me, I'm way fatter than you!' But instead I stopped myself and began to examine her figure. I had never looked at her figure, or assessed it in any way, but something about that statement made me want to. She had drawn attention to it, almost forcing me to look. I had always seen Tatiana as stunning, as you do with most of your friends; how sad and frustrating that she couldn't see it. And even sadder, that these statements of self-loathing had become so normalized in this school. How was this the norm? And even worse, how was my gut reaction to put myself down in return the norm?

Whether Tatiana was fat or not seemed irrelevant. Her weight didn't take away from her beauty. Her weight had nothing to do with how I viewed her as a person or a friend. We weren't even standing in front of a mirror. It was a door, something to be walked through, not a surface to gaze at your reflection in. Not something to be used to self-hate.

That experience stayed with me. As I grappled with my own insecurities – and my acute self-consciousness – I didn't want to be a person who continuously moaned about her body and her weight and made it a public obsession. It only made you feel worse and it drew even more attention to your insecurities. My internal battles were far from being won, and while I couldn't control what I thought of my body, I could control what I said.

# 18

## Can I change things?

Each year at St Keyes, a team of 'enterprising' girls in the sixth form would organize an ambitious charity fundraiser. As an extra-curricular activity, however, 'Young Enterprise', as it was called, had grown stale and predictable. The girls were no longer especially enterprising and the event made very little money. When it came time for girls in my year to sign up, only eleven of us were interested – a smaller number than ever. This seemed to predict that our prospects for raising money weren't so favourable.

At the first meeting, we all sat down in a conference room to listen to two supervising teachers explain how the project worked. The logistics of setting up a company were discussed, then we were told to elect a board of directors and fill a variety of available positions, from operating manager to financial manager.

I knew which position I wanted: managing director.

This was a long shot, since there were far more popular girls in the room – and five of us wanted the top job. A vote had to be held. My hope was to apply and wind up with a lower position, deputy managing director, which was given to the second runner-up. But even that seemed unlikely.

Each of the five of us was asked to give a one-minute presentation – and make a case for why we'd make the best leader.

'My father started a company when he was twenty years old,' one girl began, 'so needless to say, business has been the topic of conversation around the dinner table since I was born. I even had to do a presentation to convince him to buy me a bicycle. I know the language. I know the process. I will lead you to success.'

A second girl stood up. Lisa had always been a popular girl: beautiful, wealthy and sporty – the trifecta that guaranteed acceptance and domination at St Keyes. But after Year 11, quite a few members of her popular clique had departed the school, which had grown mellower and nicer in their absence. And now Lisa, used to her posse of mean girls, had been thrown into the mix with the rest of us. It was evident from the entitled speech she gave at Young Enterprise that she was having a hard time adjusting.

'Well, who wouldn't want me?' she said with utmost confidence. 'I'm fun, I'm already Head of House, so you know people love me. And I can bully the younger girls into donating start-up money.'

I was nervous when it was my time to speak. I couldn't

think of how to begin, or what to say. But as soon as I stood to address the ten other girls, I talked to them the way I'd talk to anyone – honestly and directly. I admitted that I didn't have much leadership experience, apart from having been the director of a school play the year before, but I told them I had really enjoyed that experience. 'I don't really know what else to say,' I went on, 'other than I think I would make a great managing director and vote for me if you think I would too.'

The self-satisfied expressions on my rivals' faces told me I'd botched it – and been too modest. But I hoped for the best when the two supervisors departed the room to count the votes of the six girls who weren't running. When they returned, one of them made an announcement.

'Well, the vote was unanimous,' she said. 'Michelle, you are our managing director.'

There are no words to describe how shocked I was. One of the supervisors continued to announce the other positions and when she was finished, she asked me to run the rest of the meeting. I stood again, this time before a whiteboard, and felt in my element, as if I'd been conducting meetings all my life.

We would throw a fashion show, we all decided, and the proceeds from the ticket sales would go to charity. We chose a name for our company: Enigma. After talking with the supervisor at the end of the meeting, I left the room. Poppy, a new friend of mine who was on the team, was waiting for me outside.

'Congratulations, managing director!' she cheered, and

gave me a hug. 'You were very official in there! So proud of you!'

'But I don't understand it,' I said. 'I couldn't have given a worse pitch.'

'It wasn't about the pitch,' Poppy explained. 'It was about your personality. You aren't popular and you aren't a loser – which means you aren't going to become power-happy like Lisa would and you aren't going to be a push-over either.'

My low-key reputation had finally worked in my favour. And I continued to run with it – deciding immediately to change the selection process for the fashion show models, and make it much more inclusive. In past years, when fashion shows were thrown at school, they'd become popularity contests with a parade of the prettiest and skinniest girls wearing unattainably expensive clothes. As managing director, I had the opportunity to throw a very different event. First of all, we could ask the local department store to loan us much more affordable clothes, rather than only high fashion. We could also ask for donations of clothing from British designers. It was going to be a fashion show of clothes that the girls could actually purchase and wear. This set us up for even bigger profits.

I began addressing all 500 girls at school assemblies to promote the event, and quickly learned that every single girl wanted to be a model. For many, it was a childhood dream to walk down a runway. I just wanted to be sure we made our selections fairly. Five members of our team, including me, sat on the selection committee and watched while the applicants poured in, from the youngest girls, still eleven years old, nervous and shy, to the girls who were a year older than us. Rather than selecting models based on appearance and popularity, I looked for unusual faces, diversity, uniqueness, personality – including girls of all shapes and sizes – and instantly disliked any signs of arrogance. My feeling was that a diverse range of girls might impact the warped culture of the school, where the skinniest and usually the meanest girls were rewarded with the most praise and status. The previous fashion shows had always been entrenched with body envy, but this was the prime opportunity to prove that every type of body was beautiful.

I also placed a ban on girls who were rude, arrogant or acted cool. 'We're not going to work with brats.' I wanted to make a point that while being mean was accepted as the norm within our school, it wouldn't be in our fashion show.

After we finalized the list of models, we invited the youngest male teacher at the school, Mr Adams, to be our host. A gap-year teacher who had graduated from a nearby boys' school, he was the heart-throb of the school and would surely boost ticket sales. Then we had to find another teacher to share in the hosting duties. This proved harder than we thought; most refused out of a fear of public speaking, which seemed ironic given that they spent most of their days speaking in front of groups of people.

'Oh, Mrs Wright will do it!' one girl called out.

'She loves the attention!' another said.

An echo of agreement came from the rest of the team.

'Fine,' I consented, 'but I'm not going to speak to her. Someone else will have to do it.'

'No, it has to be you,' the girls insisted. 'You're managing director, after all. And you need to see her to book the hall for the event – only you can do that. So either way you might as well cross both off at the same time.'

If anything, Mrs Wright had become an even more prominent figure in my life over the years at St Keyes. She had taught me every single year thus far – which was extremely unusual – and a number of extracurricular activities had led to more contact, in person and online. I saw her weekly at Summer Fete meetings, and this year in particular, she was my teacher for Critical Thinking. I had also been appointed as Community Concerns Officer. The role meant I was in charge of anything to do with the charities that the school supported, which unfortunately resulted in me being in close proximity to Mrs Wright for the frequent charity committee meetings that took place.

It wasn't unusual to see my inbox overflowing with emails from her on a variety of topics. Sometimes it felt as though my hatred for her was securely locked away in a box in my mind and I had it under control – or thought I did – and I would almost forget the incident from years before.

But she found ways to remind me, as if she were testing my memory, and my will.

'You know, Michelle,' she'd say, 'every time I look at

you I think of that weak, fragile little girl who collapsed on the floor that day, and I can't believe you're standing there, right before my very eyes, so capable. Who would have thought that that little girl would be an officer one day?'

Her timing was impeccable. She chose to make these 'encouraging' statements in a moment of celebration and pride, taking away from the accolade and yanking me back to the worst memory I held at that school. The worst memory I had, full stop.

I dreamed of being alone in a room with her, and telling her off. I imagined that she would apologize profusely and cry. One childish revenge fantasy involved waiting until the final day of school, then punching her and telling her exactly what I thought of her. This fantasy was encouraged by an experience that Esme had with Miss Naylor. Our housemistress had never seemed very supportive of Esme – to the point of actively dismissing her. After years of enduring this, Esme had confronted Miss Naylor in a private moment, unleashing a torrent of accusations of misdeeds and injustices that had left Miss Naylor apologetic and in tears.

Hearing this story empowered and emboldened me. My day would come. My moment of confrontation with Mrs Wright would be sweet – but for now I held it in.

I stood outside her door and peeked in, to check that she wasn't in a meeting. Mrs Wright was sitting at her desk behind her computer screen, typing away. Her body looked particularly angular and stiff, and her face looked even more wrinkly than usual. The white walls around her were adorned with the classic landscape paintings that were hanging all over the school – bucolic scenes of English countryside, dotted with stonewalls, haystacks and the occasional pergola or gazebo.

I knocked, and her lonely face perked up when she saw me. She waved me inside.

'Of course, I would be delighted! How kind of you to ask,' she responded to my suggestion that she host the fashion show. 'And along with Mr Adams – what a strapping young chap – we'll look fabulous together! You know, Michelle, every time I look at you I'm reminded of that feeble, weak little girl who was constantly ill and I'm just so proud to see how you've flourished. Who knew you'd be standing here, managing director and the School Community Concerns Officer nonetheless!'

I plastered a fake smile on my face, produced an artificial laugh, simply thanked her and quickly left her room. Next on the list, I had to report to Miss Naylor, who was in charge of the school swimming programme for autistic children that we had decided to donate the fashion show proceeds to. She was delighted with this news – 'How lovely of you! That's fabulous!' – then, just as I was leaving, she stopped me and said, 'It's funny you should mention Mrs Wright: I was just talking to her today about you. We are both so proud of you, and she mentioned something that I thought you might like to know.'

My heart began to pound. For a second it crossed my

mind that perhaps Mrs Wright had confessed her misdeeds and abuse years before. Maybe she was consumed by guilt – or concern about delayed legal action. But my imagination had gone off in the wrong direction.

'Mrs Wright told me you were only one vote away from being chosen as prefect,' Miss Naylor explained.

Being picked to be prefect was a life aim and dream for the girls at our school – something that could dramatically boost your university applications, but a goal that I had always felt was unattainable for me. You had to be voted in by the girls in your year as well as the teachers. Now, while it was nice to learn this news, it was also frustrating. *Only one vote away!* It was so like Mrs Wright to relay a compliment with a dark side. Something I would rather not have known.

I had started to keep a tally of these kinds of comments in my head – the times Mrs Wright made me feel bad while she pretended to be saying something good. And I realized that my revenge had already begun – with my leadership position at the fashion show, where girls of all shapes and sizes and races would model, and then, at the end, when I would lead my entire team down the catwalk for the final bow. And there would be Mrs Wright, handing me the microphone at the end of the night. In front of 200 parents and 500 girls, I would feel as powerful as I had ever felt in my life.

It was tempting to contemplate telling her off right there, with my words broadcasting through the loudspeakers. I could tell my story – and make a public demand for an apology. These fantasies would continue to play in my head, but no – it was better to wait until graduation day. Finally, I would make her feel as bad as she had made me feel all those years ago.

# 19

## How long could I keep hiding my scars?

At St Keyes, Oxbridge was the ultimate goal. Every single girl was driven to academic success: attaining the gold-merit status of being accepted into either Oxford or Cambridge – even if it meant mental breakdowns from the pressure and grind of continuous tests and mocks, routinely overdosing on caffeine, escalated bickering and competitiveness with classmates and working until all hours of the night (now that we didn't have allocated bedtimes).

This unhealthy high-wire act took over the last eighteen months of St Keyes for a majority of us. Of the ninety girls in my year, only three girls had the strength to deviate from the crowd. They weren't applying. I have to confess that I admired them. I dreamed about joining their bandwagon and becoming the fourth. I knew that I didn't want to go, I knew I would hate it, and more importantly I was unsure I could stand the academic pressure of working at this intensity for two more years – but at the same time I didn't want to be judged by my peers.

Not applying to Oxbridge was seen as an admission that you weren't smart enough; I feared that judgement and underestimated my ability to go against the crowd and resist the norm. And maybe I still had something to prove. My parents were excited for me and had contacted St Keyes to discuss my application. How could I possibly let them down? The problem was, my grades leading into final exams that year had suffered with me taking a greater interest in my extracurriculars, whether it was running Enigma or being an officer and in charge of all charity functions at the school.

I was in my last year in Rodin House so it was fitting that Miss Naylor was the person who came to my aid in the last month before my departure, almost as repentance for all the past body-shaming comments. She looked at all my courses, the material I needed to cover, and planned out every hour of every day for the following two weeks – exactly which module and which subject I would be studying at every second of the day. 'You will cancel anything that you don't need to do,' she advised me. 'Everyone will understand; getting your grades up are your priority. Stop spending time socializing. You will either be in lessons or in your room studying, and that is it.'

Miss Naylor could be seen to be an evil person but while her strict rules were annoying and at times suffocating, it mattered to me that she cared. This was rare compared to the other housemistresses, and I believed it was in these moments that she showed her true self. And her plan for my academic rehabilitation worked far better than her attempts to get me to diet. By the time I looked up from my books and emerged from social isolation, I had attained not only three As in my AS levels, but all my grades were above ninety-seven per cent – which set me up nicely for straight As the following year, and forced the school to amend my predicted grades which in turn boosted my university applications. My parents were thrilled. Oxford was now within reach.

St Keyes was so invested in our success in these interviews, and in maintaining its stellar reputation, that they brought in an external examiner whose sole job was to conduct mock interviews. The idea was that we would make mistakes and practise, then perform better in the real setting. And hopefully this would help us to relax, as we'd all heard the myths.

The Oxbridge interview questions were supposedly bizarre and unpredictable. One girl was apparently handed a rock in her Oxford interview and told to do something interesting with it. When she threw the rock out of the window, she won immediate acceptance at the school. A quick look at Oxford's website included sample interview questions such as, 'Why do human beings have two eyes?' and 'What is "normal" for humans?' Your answers were supposed to demonstrate how you think.

I did my practice interview with my psychology teacher,

Mrs Meyer. We had a comfortable relationship so I didn't experience the pre-interview jitters.

'You look calm,' she remarked as soon as I sat down. 'Well then, let's get started.'

I nodded.

'Why do you want to do psychology?' she asked.

It was the most obvious question of all and I had rehearsed the answer repeatedly. But now, directly facing Mrs Meyer, I was suddenly tongue-tied.

She stared at me, as if counting the seconds.

'Hmmm,' I answered. 'Well, I don't know. I guess I like religious studies and I guess that's quite similar and it's all about thinking.' I continued to ramble, growing more and more inarticulate while Mrs Meyer looked at me as if I wasn't speaking English. I groped around for my prepared answer – about how the things I'd seen in the hospital had caused me to want to dedicate my life to helping others – but it now seemed totally inadequate.

'Michelle, what are you doing?' Mrs Meyer finally interrupted.

'What do you mean?' I asked, feigning confusion. 'Anyway, are you allowed to interrupt me while I'm talking, as if you know me?'

'Well,' she replied, 'first of all, don't start with "I don't know". And second of all, you have the most incredible and unique reason to be studying psychology. Why aren't you talking about it? Why are you lying?'

Lying? Was I?

'Do you expect me to divulge my entire life story?'

I asked. 'I don't want to get into university on the basis of pity. I should be accepted on my intellect.'

'It's not about pity,' she explained. 'It's about giving the real reason why you have so much passion for the subject.'

The conversation continued, a brief back and forth. Then we restarted the interview and Mrs Meyer asked me the question again. But as soon as I began to explain myself and talk more personally, I burst into tears.

Worried, Mrs Meyer eased off and I found excuses to leave. Time was up. 'Don't worry, I'll just wing it on the day of the interview,' I explained as I rushed out. 'I'm late for my next lesson anyway.'

As I walked back to my house, I tried to comprehend what had just happened. In the past, when the subject of my health came up, it had been easy to skate on the surface. The real story of my surgeries and scars had been playing only in my head all these years; they had never been voiced. I hadn't realized that I had never actually vocalized this story that played on repeat in my brain. I hadn't realized until I was sitting in that room, in that moment, how hard it would be to describe in person. And now, just thinking about it filled me with unbearable, excruciating sadness. I was on the edge of panic.

A similar feeling had come over me the year before this, almost foretelling this situation. During a general studies lesson, the subject of abortion had been raised. The teacher had explained that there were certain cases in which a woman who was pregnant was allowed to abort a baby at full term – due to the severity of the baby's health, or due to a threat to the mother's life.

In a moment of curiosity, I raised my hand.

'What kind of condition do you have to have to abort at full term?' I asked. 'Like, how severe does it have to be?'

'Well, you probably won't know what this is,' the teacher explained, 'but there's a condition called hydrocephalus. If the baby has that, you can abort up to the day before it's expected to be born.'

At the mention of hydrocephalus, tears began rolling down my face. By the time she had finished the sentence, I was crying uncontrollably. In my embarrassment, I got up and squeezed past all the girls in the row and ran out the door and into the corridor. Behind me I could hear the teacher asking the class what had happened – whether it was something she had said. I was hyperventilating by then, leaning against a wall, hunched over, trying to calm myself. When I looked up, the teacher appeared before me.

'Michelle, I'm so sorry,' she said, placing her hand on my shoulder, attempting to console me. 'Do you know someone who has it? I had no idea.'

'Me,' I muttered through tears, my head in my hands. 'I have it.'

'But you're so normal,' she said, 'no one would ever know. A baby wouldn't be aborted in a situation like yours. It would have to be a much more severe case.'

The word 'normal' stung. What was normal? Did my condition and surgeries make me *not* normal? Or could I stay normal, as long as they remained hidden and I acted as if they never affected me?

When I returned to class, the room fell silent and nothing was mentioned. Later, Miss Naylor was informed about the incident and checked on me. When she asked if I was OK I reassured her that it was nothing. I said that I couldn't really explain what had happened.

But privately, to myself, I had a good guess. Being an unexpected pregnancy, I wondered if my mum had considered an abortion. Did she know about my hydrocephalus in the womb? If she had, would she have wanted me? There were so many unanswered questions about my life – things I'd never thought to ask my parents, things I'd never thought to ask myself. Surviving and thriving at St Keyes had required forward motion. I looked ahead, not behind. I moved on, and didn't question what was in the past. And, just as I had learned in the hospital, I tried to stay on the positive, sunny side of things – upbeat and funny. The irony wasn't lost on me that I had spent the last seven years planning to be a psychologist, but I couldn't be farther away from the actual practice of it. How would I ever talk to other people about their scars and fears and bad memories if I couldn't talk about my own?

My real Oxford interview didn't go much better than the practice one. It was a bitterly cold December morning when I walked into a cosy university room with shelves overflowing with books, and a panel of three people sitting in front of me – two men and a woman. Before I had a chance to even approach the table, or sit down, one of the men asked:

'Cube root of sixty-four?'

I hesitated for a moment, alarmed by the abrupt nature of the question. Then I replied, 'Eight,' before realizing, a second later, that I had responded with the square root and not the cube root. Before I had a chance to correct myself, another question was fired off. I still hadn't even had the chance to sit down.

'Log one hundred?' the woman asked. I fumbled for an answer. In my maths class at St Keyes, we hadn't gotten to studying logs yet, although I figured a guess would be better than simply saying I didn't know.

'Ten,' I said, quite certain of my inaccuracy.

'You can sit down now,' the woman responded. 'And for the record, you got both of those wrong.'

The intimidating questions continued – as did my fumbling, nervous responses and second-guesses. An hour later, in the second interview I was handed a psychology article to read, followed by a series of questions about the statistical tools used to analyse the data, then an abstract puzzle. Four double-sided cards with an assortment of letters and corresponding numbers on each side were held up and I was asked to predict which card would hold a certain letter.

'No, you don't understand the question,' one interviewer pointed out.

In our practice interviews at St Keyes, we had been warned about this – that interviewers might try to trip us up, or persuade us to retract our answer to see how confident we were. We were advised to give an answer and stand firm.

'Yes, I do,' I replied with utmost confidence. 'It's the right answer.'

We continued to argue back and forth, before I realized that I had misheard the letter 'E' for the number three and that I had, in fact, been wrong the entire time.

I went from one failure to another with each subsequent interview. And I never discussed my true reasons for wanting to study psychology, other than my fascination with the Stanford prison experiment – a famous study of inmates done by psychologist Philip Zimbardo. I had found it fascinating how environment could change people so significantly, that upstanding citizens, when told to pretend to be inmates, started to act accordingly. More alarmingly, the participants who were told to be guards, within twenty-four hours had let the power go to their head, completely forgetting that this was an experiment. What fascinated me most about the study was how much it reminded me of St Keyes – how, once we were within a system, we all just learned to conform.

My rejection came as no surprise to me. 'Thank you for accepting our invitation for interview. I am writing now to let you know that after careful consideration, it has not been possible to offer you a place at Magdalen College.'

'They must have made a mistake,' Mum said in disbelief. 'Call them back and check that they sent you the right letter.'

'It's because they didn't give you time to read the article beforehand!' my dad complained. 'They need to give you a fair chance.'

Days later, my parents were still in denial but I had moved on. In the future, I would be free of the stressed-out hyper-competitive treadmill. At least wherever I ended up, whatever university would have me, I was going to be able to have a life outside of my studies – perhaps even a social life?

That's when this tight pain in my chest would set in. I imagined myself having balance in my life, and all kinds of new friends, but all of it felt tainted by pressure and fear. Every time I imagined meeting my room-mate for the first time or talking to a boy, I felt a wave of panic inside. How would I tell them about myself, and my life? How long could I keep hiding my scars?

# 20

## And how do you feel about that?

It wasn't appropriate for a St Keyes girl to admit having too many feelings, or confusion about them – much less see a psychologist. Often, any vulnerability would be used against you, but not before being quietly reserved for the next fight or used as fodder for the next gossip session. At worst, confessions about your 'issues' would raise the threat of being shipped off to The Priory in the dark of night. These extreme measures were only for the serious cases, when girls were wasting away into ghosts from trying to get thinner, or if they had been suffering from depression after the constant workload had grown too much, or perhaps begun wearing bracelets up to their elbows to disguise self-harm.

Say nothing. Feel nothing. That was the path to fitting in.

There was a woman you could 'talk to' though, if you were in emotional distress – a school 'counsellor'. She was called simply 'Harriet' – perhaps their way of trying to make her appear more relatable, but an informality that immediately reduced her status at St Keyes. The girls all looked down on therapy, on the premise that only 'crazy people' needed it. I had never once heard a girl refer to Harriet seriously, or warmly, or with any sense of respect. She was solely the subject of gossip and a punchline of jokes.

Remarks such as, 'You're being rude, leave me alone!' would be responded to with, 'Boo-hoo, go see Harriet and cry about it.' She was associated with St Keyes flops and failures; girls who didn't have the emotional fortitude to endure the slings and arrows that the *Lord-of-the-Flies* school environment delivered.

To make matters worse, everyone knew where Harriet's office was – in a very public spot, directly opposite the medical centre, which meant that girls seen coming and going were whispered about. The reason for a visit was assumed to be one of four things: anorexia, bulimia, depression or self-harm. Or so I thought. But when I mentioned to one of the more compassionate girls, a relatively new friend in my new house, that I had been unable to talk about my surgeries or scars during my Oxford interview, or in my mock interview with Mrs Meyer – or even to describe why I wanted to study psychology – she told me about another girl in our year who had been to see Harriet about all kinds of things, from exam stress to friendship issues.

'She's paid by the school to just sit there and listen,' my new friend said. 'What harm would it be to go and try to talk to her?'

I was sitting in front of my computer and staring at my application for the University of Bristol when, instead, I opened up my email and composed a letter to Harriet. I kept the title of the email vague. And I sent it from a private account so the school would have no record of it. I didn't even sign it with my name.

My appointment was scheduled for 2 pm on a Thursday, which was completely inconvenient. It was my final year at St Keyes, which meant our year group was now living together in a new house called Highgrove. This was separated into ten smaller houses each comprising ten girls – largely divided by our friendship groups. Thursday afternoons were a blissful, sacred time. I had no classes after 10 am and would spend the rest of the day sitting in the kitchen as my friends passed in and out between their lessons; then around lunchtime we usually gathered to discuss the events of the day while baking brownies and sharing them. These afternoons were among the best times that I had had at the school, when university applications had been sent off and a more relaxed atmosphere prevailed. It pained me to imagine missing out on them.

I also knew it would be hard to step out undetected.

Thursday came, and 2 pm approached. I was sitting nervously at the kitchen table with my laptop, trying to sneak through the school's firewall to get access to Facebook, with a few of my friends pottering around, making their lunch. I looked up and noticed there wasn't long to go until my appointment, when the bell rang and more people filed in. The kitchen was full by this point, both the cooking area and the large table we all sat at. With a new version of Sims out, my friends had become obsessed and I secretly hoped this would distract them from my absence.

*Should I say I have a squash lesson?* No – some of the girls knew my squash lesson was on a Tuesday. Rather than offer an excuse, I decided to just leave the room without a mention, in the middle of a conversation, as if I were simply going to the bathroom. But as I pulled open the door, Charlotte stopped mid-sentence.

'Where are you going?'

'Oh, didn't I tell you? I have a driving lesson,' I replied.

'How can you have a driving lesson?' she asked. 'Your provisional licence hasn't even arrived.'

'Oh yeah, it came this morning,' I said. 'Didn't I tell you?'

Then Poppy perked up – suddenly curious. 'How did you book a driving lesson on the same day you got your licence?' she asked. It was a sensible enough question.

Clearly I hadn't thought this through.

'Why are you guys being so annoying?' I replied. 'I'm going to a driving lesson. I'm going to be late. Bye.' I darted out of the room quickly, knowing I had just raised more suspicion. But I had larger things to worry about – like, what the hell was I going to talk about with Harriet?

I walked down the corridor to her office. Across the way, I saw the school nurse moving around inside the medical centre – the location of so many bad memories of my earlier years – and upstairs, Rodin House – a place I was so happy to have left.

It wasn't quite 2 pm, so I hovered outside Harriet's door until I realized that my hovering was becoming noticed by the nurses. I ducked into the toilet, where I counted down the minutes until it was time to knock on Harriet's door.

'Hi, nice to meet you,' she said as I entered. All the older women at St Keyes had the same sickening posh drawl that filled me with instant dread. But Harriet smiled in a motherly way. Her nature seemed gentler than most in the school; she had a manner that was almost a stereotype of what a counsellor should have.

'Hi, I'm Michelle,' I said, unsure what to say next – or where to begin.

'How are you doing?' she started. It was such an open-ended question, but led naturally to me trying to explain what I was doing there. So I sat down and began to recount the events of my mock interview with Mrs Meyer and how it had revealed my fear of talking about my operations.

And then, as I began to tell the story, almost on cue, I started to cry.

I struggled, trying to collect myself enough to explain my medical past in a concise way – like what I had been told about my hospital stays when I was a baby. Then I moved onto my first memory of the surgery when I was seven, and finally reached the events I feared most – my first year at St Keyes, when I was eleven.

I talked nonstop. Hardly a pause of any kind. It was partially out of awkwardness and discomfort, and partially because this was truly the first time I had described the entire parade of procedures and conditions.

When I caught my breath, Harriet intervened. 'And how do you feel about that?'

My running monologue continued, in which I revealed – in a burst – my deepest concerns about university. Wouldn't I be meeting all kinds of new people who would be curious about this? I didn't specifically mention boys, taking off my clothes, being seen naked, or sex, but she probably had enough of an imagination to guess that this was behind my fears.

As she nodded along sympathetically, tears continued to stream down my face. All of a sudden, two hours had passed.

'Well,' she said with a soft smile, 'that's all we have time for today. Same time next week?'

As I walked out, I admitted to myself that I had warped the story slightly, avoiding the incidents with Mrs Wright and shying away from topics that were the hardest to talk about – namely the moment that I had died and been revived. I was afraid of being pitied, which I hated, or even worse, not believed. But the process of speaking out loud about my experiences – even if it was an abbreviated version – somehow meant these things had actually happened. It was all true. And it was all part of my past. That alone seemed like enough. Maybe, I surmised, the real achievement of going to therapy was the ability to just get there, in essence admitting that you needed help.

I saw Harriet again the following week, and the one

after that. It became easier in a way, because I realized that what I shared was completely up to me. The more sessions I attended, the more real my problems felt. But they were also beginning to feel too deep to uncover – or really explore. The more obvious it became that my hospital experience had affected me, the more detached I became – and scared. I had built a wall around my saddest feelings. This wall was tall and compartmentalized a part of me that I didn't want to see, and a part of me I didn't recognize. The tears that came out in Harriet's sessions didn't feel like the real me. The real me was not a sad person. The real me didn't cry – not even when I watched *The Notebook*. I was high-energy. I was positive. That was who I wanted to be, liked to be and chose to be. If I pulled out even one of the bricks of the wall to peek inside, it could lead to all the bricks tumbling down, destroying the parts of me that I liked, introducing me to a world of misery that I could potentially never escape. Who would I be then, if I didn't have my walls?

And besides, I had always been told that I was lucky. It hadn't escaped my awareness that there were kids still in the ICU. Once I left, there was another ill child to replace me. Once others left, there were even more to replace them. Those floors were never vacant. The beds were always being used. Surgeries were happening each and every day and I was lucky that I wasn't having them. To focus on my experience, or feel sad about it, would not only be selfish, but disrespectful to all the children who were still in hospital today – or worse, didn't survive. And to all the parents who had to go through something like that. They were the ones with real pain, heartache, insurmountable loss and sadness. A loss that I found hard to even comprehend. The least I could do was keep them in my thoughts and stop thinking about myself so much.

With each week, I found it harder and harder to attend the session, and my conversations with Harriet became less and less relevant. On my way to her office, I would tell myself that this was going to be the week that I delved courageously into the pain I suspected was still down there, along with all my memories of hospitalizations and probably the sadness and confusion that I knew should be there. Instead, I discussed petty friendship dramas or I exaggerated stories about how debilitated I was from homework and academic stress. In reality, my friendships were great and there was next to no schoolwork to be done. My grades from the previous year had guaranteed me a place at Bristol, my chosen university. There was truly nothing relevant to complain about – yet I always found things.

No matter what we discussed, one fact was guaranteed: from the moment I sat down, I would begin crying and I wouldn't stop until the moment I got up to leave. Running out of stories, and reasons for crying, I began to cancel my sessions, telling Harriet that I had fallen ill or that a lesson had been rescheduled – and eventually stopping therapy altogether. I claimed that I needed those extra two hours in my week to focus solely on my exams. What was the point of all this talk with Harriet, I told myself, when I was leaving the school for good in less than a month?

# 21

## Am I an adult now?

On my last morning at St Keyes, I woke up in my narrow single bed and looked around the room. My eyes landed on the remaining photographs on my bulletin board. While packing up the night before, I had left them in place – unable to bear the thought of sleeping with blank institutional walls on my very last night. The bulletin board was adorned with my memories, images of the Rodin girls from the earlier years, and of my friends at Highgrove. They showed school trips, holiday parties, candid moments in our dorms and a few funnier selfies from the days when we were bored while studying. Each image brought back memories of conversations, and even arguments.

My days at the school had not been as happy as my pinboard reflected. Mostly it had been an obstacle course, another kind of survival mode. In order to go on, I'd had to insist that I was OK. Not just OK, but *lucky*. And, of course, I was.

It's my nature to be stubborn, to look forward. To get up and go. Each year I had remained at the school had proven the law of physics: a body in motion will stay in motion.

And now, here I was, feeling sad about leaving. St Keyes had been an essential part of my life – it had constituted seven years of it – and lying there in my bed, staring up at the photos, I couldn't believe the last day had come.

Boxes and bags filled the floor around me, full of all the stuff that I had accumulated over the years.

I climbed out of bed and began digging through the boxes, looking for my makeup bag. In the majority of the time I had spent at school, this bag had only surfaced for special occasions when I'd needed to make an effort. At St Keyes, girls who wore makeup to classes were laughed at. Who were they trying to impress? Our clothes had gotten grubbier over the years too. As the oldest girls in the school, we were allowed to wear our own things and we all pushed the boundaries of how little effort we could make. Tracksuit bottoms and oversized hoodies had become our new uniforms, along with the occasional pyjama day when you overslept and had to rush to chapel.

But today, we had all been told to make an effort. The night before, I had even blow-dried my hair to tame the frizz. For once, my morning fight with my hairbrush would be worth it – my lasting impression on St Keyes, memorialized in all the graduation pictures.

All the graduating girls had been instructed to wear a straight skirt and blazer to the ceremony. Like most of the other girls, I had spent the last two weeks finding just the right ones – a black blazer and matching pencil skirt. I paired this with a bright red silk blouse to add a little bit of personality to the outfit, and then added a perfect gold necklace and a pair of black kitten heels. (I'd had to get approval for my outfit from the housemistress.)

Surfacing from my room, I found that my friends were already in various states of dress, gathering in the kitchen and filling it with laughter.

My friendship group was kind and caring. Laura, Poppy, Eloise and Charlotte were an eclectic group, but were warm and supportive. Before leaving for boarding school when I was eleven, my mum had told me it would be like 'one big sleepover', and that's exactly what it felt like now, just as I was leaving. It had taken me five years of battling at Rodin House before I'd found the kind of friends I'd always longed for. We still fought, but the fights were pettier and the apologies faster. The kitchen was our gathering place; it was where we had our rituals – staying up until 2 am baking, usually brownies, which we stood around and forked into our mouths while we chatted.

It was where we'd planned our own muck-up day, when the departing girls played practical jokes on the school. Over the last seven years, the pranks had become tamer with a crackdown on what would be tolerated, so our year decided to keep it pleasant. Our house was responsible for decorating the houses in the main school building

– Rodin and Tate – and we adorned our designated area of destruction like a fairytale crime scene. The staircases became a giant beanstalk and we drew human print-marks, while in other areas girls painted the walls with a Banksy-style mural – a project so artistically done that the school welcomed it – and hung all the school clocks from the trees in an *Alice in Wonderland* style. We spent the last two days baking cupcakes and distributing them throughout the corridors, and going into the exam hall to hang a banner saying 'Good Luck' to cheer up the younger girls sitting their GCSEs – and leaving cookies on each of their tables.

It had taken weeks of planning, with everybody coming together in unity to present our final goodbye. We dressed up as Pac-Man and rode around the school on scooters with water pistols, soaking any younger girl walking past us and taking over the chapel sermon in a scene that wasn't too dissimilar to the movie *Sister Act*. We organized a special Chinese meal with the catering staff (everyone's favourite meal, usually served on Chinese New Year) and serenaded everyone in the dining room with a flash mob, as the TV show *Glee* had hit its peak popularity that year. We took over the school assembly, putting in a few jokes at the younger girls' and teachers' expense before airing our version of the *Mean Girls* trailer, St Keyes style. We had left our mark on the school, and it was a pleasant one. The teachers were happy and the girls were happy; we'd done it in a tasteful, smart way, indicative of our year group.

I knew I would miss the closeness, the complaining, the constant proximity to my friends and the camaraderie. I had grown so comfortable around these girls that, two weeks before, I'd even told them about my sessions with Harriet. And rather than the judgement and harsh criticism that I'd expected, they responded with kindness and curiosity. They weren't appalled; they were fascinated. *Why did you do that? What was bothering you?*

'You know,' Laura said, 'you've never actually told me what happened to you in hospital.'

The kitchen went silent. Laura had started at St Keyes in sixth form – so it made sense that she might not have any idea of what my childhood had been like, and the health issues I'd endured. The rest of the girls in the room were a random collection – mostly ones I'd known for ages, some since the first year, like Eloise.

'Oh, it's boring,' I said, reflexively wanting to change the subject. 'And I'm sure Eloise and the other girls know the story already. I'll tell you another time.'

'Actually, we don't,' Eloise interjected. We'd known each other for six years, but hadn't been close until that last year. Still, it shocked me to realize that she hadn't heard much about the story – even third- or fourth-hand. I had never really voiced it aloud.

I dove in and began my story, dialling down the drama but keeping in the humorous parts, encouraged when the room exploded in laughter at my descriptions. I told them about the nits in my hair, the windmills I made while spending my days in bed, the dogs I played with, and how each person in the ICU had left a lasting impression on me: the doctors, nurses, psychologists, and the children who'd died. When I backtracked to my account of fainting in Mrs Wright's classroom, one girl cried out that she remembered being there, the shock of it, and for some peculiar reason, how I'd been lying with my head down on the desk, softened by the little pillow that I'd made in our textiles class.

The girls were loving and supportive, exclaiming, 'Michelle! No! I can't believe you had to go through that!' I felt buoyed and stronger – and for a few days afterwards, I felt a small glimmer of hope that I would be able to explain all these difficult things someday when I tried to make new friends at university. But each day, as the end of school approached, and university loomed, my worries worsened.

It had taken me almost seven years to find these friends. How long would it take at university? My older sister had tried to reassure me, telling me that your university years were 'the best years of your life'. But that made me worry more. My sister, being twelve years older, had always felt more like a second mum and I valued her advice deeply but this statement felt like it added to my feelings of expectation and pressure. What if I didn't meet anyone I liked? And if I did meet friends, how would I tell them about my operations? How would I bring it up?

At the leaving ceremony, I spotted my parents in the front row, waving and smiling. I hadn't seen them in more than two months. There was nothing I wanted more than to run up to them and hug them; but instead I was stuck with formalities – being ushered into a row of Rodin girls, organized in alphabetical order. Since moving to Highgrove, the now eleven girls from my year in Rodin were rarely all together but it seemed fitting for the last day since they were the girls who were my everyday friends for so long.

The girls had gathered again, all dressed and ready, to say our goodbyes, or try to, before taking some pictures to remember the day by. I had been pleased when, joining the rest of our year in the common room for the last outfit check, the head girl had bumped into me, apologized, and then done a double-take. 'Michelle? Whoa. You look so different, I barely recognized you!'

*I liked that she said 'different' and not 'better'. So often women believe they look better in makeup.*

We'd made our way to the grandiose hall, complete with a balcony near the ceiling and wooden arches across the roof, and adorned with paisley curtains in a canary yellow and blue that matched the blue carpet on the stage.

We took our seats and then, as the members of staff walked onto the stage before us, we all rose – as we had been taught on that very first day at St Keyes, and as we had done ever since, in every single class, at the beginning of every single lesson. I watched as each member of staff entered, studying them carefully. Mrs Meyer, my psychology teacher, Mrs Abbott who taught me chemistry, Mrs Garner who taught me maths, and even the staff who'd taught me in the younger years: my Spanish teacher, my geography teacher, my history teacher – all the subjects I'd been so glad to be rid of. Mrs Paulson, the headmistress, welcomed us, and allowed us to take our seats. The last few women, who held the highest positions in the school, arrived and took their places in the front row. Next to the headmistress sat Miss Naylor – my housemistress for five years – and right next to her, Mrs Wright. They wore matching pearl earrings with a pearl necklace: standard St Keyes attire.

The headmistress began. She made the customary welcome to our parents, who were now seated behind us, and went on to give a speech about the importance of this day. Then the head girl – the girl in our year that held the most power, chosen by both girls and staff – took her place and said a few choice words to inspire and motivate us about the new life that we would live. After about twenty minutes, each row of soon-to-be graduates stood and walked single-file to a spot below the stage.

Standing before everyone, waiting for my turn to receive my certificate and shake hands with the headmistress, I turned to look at the audience. I spotted my parents and smiled. I remember thinking, *Whatever you do, don't fall over*. I was wearing heels – a rare event – which made me wobble around.

I heard a name announced: 'Michelle Almond.' *I guess that's me?* The headmistress's mispronunciation of my name seemed ironic and almost apt. How many times had she said my name over the years, on the very same stage, whether it was inviting me up to speak on behalf of charities or for our fashion show? Surely my impact on the school as Community Concerns Officer was enough to at least learn my name?

I walked the four steps up to the stage, teetering, then walked across to shake hands with the headmistress. As I walked past Miss Naylor, she began clapping in an overly enthusiastic manner. Next to her was Mrs Wright.

Her smile caught my attention. It was an eerily soft expression – almost one of pride. The cruel grin was gone. I saw something softer, even gentle. I wondered if the idea of my graduating brought her relief and comfort. As long as I was still within the walls of St Keyes, I was a walking reminder of her worst failings as a teacher and human being. Did she ever flinch, just thinking of how close she came to being admonished or fired? Or perhaps being reported, stripped of her ability to teach forever?

I had entered the school as a small, thin girl lacking any style, with pink and purple glasses and my hair slicked back in a ponytail. I'd been a nervous, anxious girl who was fearful of teachers yet often overly hyper to compensate. I'd jumped on beds the very first night, irritating my room-mates. I'd been loud and vocal, sensitive, argumentative and stubborn. And I was plagued by migraines.

Yet here I was, driven by vengeance and determination, seven years later. My successes had surprised Mrs Wright, and she'd said as much each time she got a chance. But they had surprised me too. How had I done it?

False confidence had played a part. It was something of a tradition at the school. We were all taught manners, how to be polite and eloquent, how to address figures of authority, how to exist in a grown-up setting and communicate with parents and staff alike, in writing and in person. Confidence was taught indirectly, when we were put in positions of authority and responsibility. It went along with public speaking, how to give a firm handshake upon entry to a room, how to project when speaking to an audience. Regardless of your age, you were considered capable and you were treated as such.

Faking it was necessary to survival – particularly at St Keyes. My greatest fears were still alive inside me, alongside my insecurities. But, at the same time, I had created a facade that had worked. And a facade that might continue to hold up and help me.

The rest of the ceremony whizzed by, with awards handed out and everything eventually coming to a close. I found my parents afterwards and introduced them to my Rodin friends as well as my newer friends. Being half a world away, they had never met any of them.

Miss Naylor approached us, and embraced my parents. They had always been fans of Miss Naylor – knowing only about the times when she had consoled me through problems, and less so about the times when she had been the cause of them. I listened while they shared their pride over my accomplishments and my placement at Bristol. Moments later, Miss Naylor disappeared into a circle of other parents.

Then Mrs Wright appeared. I froze in place – suddenly

realizing that my parents had never met her. 'Oh, how proud we are of Michelle!' she exclaimed in that starchy voice of hers. 'Who would have thought that that tiny girl from first year would have blossomed into such a fantastic young lady? I still remember the time when you were so poorly; I'd never recognize that little thing from the vivacious girl standing before me now.'

She beamed, and placed her hand on my arm.

'Yes, we are proud,' Dad responded, a smile plastered on his face. He had always found the teachers in my school humorous, unnecessarily flamboyant, and thought their cartoonish over-the-top accents matched their ridiculous personalities. Next to him, Mum was smiling and nodding. A moment later, Mrs Wright excused herself and began talking to other parents.

'Who is that strange woman?' Dad asked.

'That was Mrs Wright,' I replied flatly, a feeling of grave disappointment rising in my chest. My sense of regret was instant and profound. For seven years I had dreamed of the day, this day, this moment, in which I could fire back and confront her – and wipe that ridiculous smile from her face. My chance for vengeance had vanished.

'What? You mean the woman who wasn't very nice to you in first year?' my mum asked. 'Who was rude to you when you were sick?'

I left my parents to join my celebrating friends, and my gaze turned to Mrs Wright again. She was nodding and smiling, shaking the hands of parents, looking pleased and uncomfortable. This was a woman who had come to St Keyes herself as a girl, met her husband at a school social here, sent her kids here, only to return and teach here, and spend most of her life inside the school walls. It seemed such an isolated existence – separated from the rest of the world. She loved describing her own glory days, telling her students that her 'St Keyes days' were the best years of her life. I kept watching her, wondering when the feelings of revenge would well up inside me again and I would stride over to her and have my say. It wasn't too late. But she looked so uncomfortable already. More than nervous, she seemed uneasy in her own skin. Without a cigarette to calm her, she seemed tense. Her blue suit was like a shield. And she seemed sad. A sense of pity washed over me.

Even at my age, I already seemed more comfortable in my own skin.

# SECTION THREE

# 22

## Do I have to ask?

The drinking game had started. Our part of the residence hall or 'block' at Bristol was a long L-shaped corridor with forty individual suites. In the middle was our living room, which we quickly nicknamed The Boardroom because it was where we convened at all hours of the day. We were all bright-eyed freshers who were just getting to know one another.

In the middle of The Boardroom was a long wooden table. There was a drinking cup in the middle, surrounded by a collection of cards. Bottles of alcohol were placed along the edges of the table, an assortment of the cheapest and strongest mixtures of spirits and fizzy drinks. We were playing 'Ring of Fire'. Each card that was chosen indicated the task we had to play, determined by the number on the card. If a two of clubs was picked, it meant you had to consume two fingers of a drink. If you picked a seven, that meant Truth or Dare.

'Your turn, pick a card,' Freddie said.

Freddie was the only person on the corridor who was studying psychology, like me. A mutual friend had introduced us once she had discovered we did the same course. But one look at this guy with broad shoulders and bulging muscles and I knew that he would probably be civil, but would never become a friend. He looked like a 'lad'. Purely based on his appearance, I figured he would definitely be in one of the sports teams – rugby, football or perhaps basketball due to his height. The initiations for these societies were infamous; these guys weren't just interested in sporting accomplishments but sexual ones as well – complete with sexist banter and binge-drinking to the point of paralysis.

My suspicions about Freddie were further supported when we spoke. He asked where I'd gone to school. I hesitated – not wanting to say. I'd been warned by several friends that just the name St Keyes would conjure a wealth of judgements and assumptions, and I should avoid talking about it at all costs. They'd said it would broadcast to one and all that I was a sheltered girl with no life experience, a boring geek, or more commonly, an acne-covered loser with no social life.

As soon as I arrived at university, I discovered that answering this question was unavoidable. It was the first thing anybody asked. Each time I was asked and replied, I waited for the fallout – and the jokes. But instead, I discovered that most people had never even heard of St Keyes, and had to ask what kind of school it was. This seemed true of many top women's schools. If only girls went there, nobody cared.

But not Freddie. His eyes lit up the instant the words 'St Keyes' came out of my mouth.

'The Virgin Megastore!' he called out. 'No prizes for guessing who's going to be going wild tonight. Doesn't everyone from your school go crazy once they're free of their restrictive parents?'

This last remark, 'restrictive parents', referred to my being half-Chinese. Admittedly, this stereotype would have been suitable for the majority of the Hong Kong girls at St Keyes, with their strict academic regimen and other academic pressures, including extra tutoring during all summer holidays – effectively making school a nonstop year-round experience. But it wasn't true of me. My parents were lenient and felt summers should be for holidays and relaxing. In any case, I chose to laugh it off. Based on my own stereotyping of him, I assumed he and I weren't going to be friends anyway.

Music blared from a tiny speaker in the corner of The Boardroom and the card game continued. The boys on our corridor had started the game, and the rest of the girls were still straggling in after completing their 'getting-ready' process. Seeing that it was going to be a long night, I grabbed one of the comfier seats, attracting the company of some new friends who perched casually on the arms of my chair while others parked on overturned bins, stacked beanbags or were sitting on the bar.

'Ace, waterfall. Guys, shut up! Waterfall.'

It was my new friend Alex that made this announce-ment, and on cue, conversations around the room stopped and we all began drinking – until we were commanded to stop. Alex was boyish and likeable, extremely extroverted and open, with a silly, charming side to him that brought out the bold side in me.

It was surprisingly easy to make friends at Bristol – a shock after the largely chilly St Keyes. Arriving on the first day, the first person I'd met was a girl called Emma, whose room was exactly opposite mine. As soon as my mum had departed, I'd pushed myself out of my comfort zone and decided to try to meet people, so I walked across the corridor and just knocked on the door, wanting to say hi to whomever was there.

A petite blonde had opened the door and looked at me with a blank stare as I introduced myself. She said her name, then closed her door again.

*My neighbour is a bitch*, I thought to myself. *Off to a great start!* But it just shows how wrong first impres-sions can be. Emma and I would become inseparable. Our corridor – V Block – quickly became a tight-knit group, even though the mix of personalities was varied. Some were academic types, some were sporty, some were even a bit difficult, yet everyone was accepting and welcoming – something I hadn't expected. You were free to be yourself, and as weird and wonderful as you pleased. And unlike at St Keyes, your quirks wouldn't be met with weird stares and judgemental looks. Instead, there were people laughing along with you. Our bond was so strong that by the middle of the year, our corridor became known as The Bermuda Triangle. Those who came for a party or a visit never left: they didn't want to.

The drinking game continued. Another card was chosen. It was an eight, which indicated a round of the game 'Never Have I Ever'. The person who selected the card had to state something that they hadn't done sexually.

'Never have I ever had a threesome!'

There were a whole lot of never-evers for me. Only two nights before, I had had my first kiss from a boy. It was at the inaugural fresher's party, for which each residence hall was allocated a particular dress code and theme. Our theme was 'Army'. So we had all donned dog tags, painted our faces with green and black stripes, and dressed in an assortment of brown, black and green attire that we had found in each other's wardrobes earlier that day.

A few tequila shots and cranberry vodkas later, and in the midst of a swirl of flashing fluorescent lights, I had turned around while dancing in a circle of girls and some-how found myself in the arms of a boy. He was tall and attractive and also wearing army gear. I began to apologize but he leaned into me and before I knew it, we were kissing.

'I'm Hugo from M Block,' he said. I kissed him again and then darted off to join my friends.

The following morning, Emma had knocked at my door and picked me up on her way to breakfast. I sat down to eat in silence, as she began chatting to a boy next to me. My headache was throbbing as I attempted to be sociable, asking if they'd enjoyed themselves the night before. After demolishing our food, Emma and I got up to leave, when the boy stopped her.

'Wait, I didn't catch your name?' he inquired, totally ignoring me.

'Oh, Emma. I'm in V Block,' she responded.

'Nice to meet you,' the boy said. 'I'm Hugo from M Block.'

My heart stopped. I couldn't remember much from the night before, but you would've thought I might at least have remembered the face of the first boy I ever kissed. I smiled at him, trying to ease over any awkward tension that I might have created.

'This is Michelle,' Emma said, nodding towards me.

'Oh, we've met,' Hugo said with a sweet smile.

Walking away after breakfast, I filled Emma in. 'Oh my god – I kissed that guy last night, and I completely forgot!'

'Hugo? He's cute. When did you kiss? I thought I was with you the whole night.' She laughed and gave me a shove.

'It was kind of my first kiss,' I admitted, slightly embarrassed.

'Well... how was it?'

'Slobbery.' I giggled as we returned to our block.

It had felt nice admitting the truth. Even better, Emma had seemed more intrigued than shocked. Jokes about being a virgin hadn't materialized, the way they would have at St Keyes. You didn't have to maintain this delicate balance between being a 'slut' and a 'prude' here. There were no judgements. Here, my friends were simply accepting.

In fact, plenty of people on my corridor were in a similar situation and made no attempt to hide it.

Another card got picked, and another round began. 'Three. Rule Master. You get to make a rule,' someone called out. It was Alex's turn again.

'Michelle has to sit with her top off for the next round,' he said with a smirk.

A number of people had had to strip already, on other nights during other drinking games. But I had managed to escape, conveniently leaving the room when names were called out. Nudity seemed to accompany many of the sexual confessions on these nights, and went along with dares like having to drink shots off of someone's belly button or having to do a strip dance.

'Oh, come on! Not fair!' I called out, hoping to argue my way out of it. 'Pick something reasonable!'

'I had to take off my top yesterday,' one of the other girls chimed in. 'So Michelle has to do it today.'

'Come on, don't make it a big deal,' Alex continued. 'It's not like we're going to be staring at you, anyway; we aren't pervs. It's not like I'm asking you to take your bra off.'

'Well you are a perv, just for asking in the first place,' I retorted. 'But fine – whatever.'

I stood to take my top off. Alex began to cheer for a few seconds, and then, as my top rose over my bare torso, he became quiet. The rest of the crowd weren't even paying attention; they'd moved onto the next person – more interested in the acceptance of the dare rather than actually watching it happen.

'Oh, I'm sorry, Michelle,' Alex stammered. 'So sorry – you don't have to… ummm, I didn't know.'

Scars. Naturally, he hadn't expected them. If he'd known about them, I'm sure he wouldn't have dared me to undress. Even I had been too drunk to consider them or to hesitate because of them. The thing I had always feared most was happening right now – and I had, for the first time in my life, forgotten about my scars. While nobody in the room had seemed to care when I took my top off, and had continued to converse among themselves, Alex's abject apology caught their attention. The room grew silent.

'I should probably explain,' I mumbled. 'It's not a big deal…'

This was certainly *not* how I'd imagined all my friends would find out.

I put my top back on and continued to explain. 'I've just had a few operations.'

'What for?'

'Operations?'

Suddenly, I was fielding questions – and for the first time in my life, people were genuinely interested in my response. Each answer led to three more questions. Didn't that hurt? How long were you in hospital? How many surgeries? With a few pre-med students in the room, there were even questions about physiological technicalities and a discussion of the word 'hydrocephalus'. The collaborative effort that went into explaining my medical procedures made me feel comforted, as the room listened in awe and, inevitably, after a few minutes, everyone got distracted and the conversation moved on. And then, thankfully, the night went on as if nothing happened. The game continued.

Alex pulled me to one side. 'I'm sorry. I feel really bad, I didn't mean to out you like that.'

To be honest, I was grateful. It was a relief to not be hiding this secret – and worrying how everyone would find out. All that anxiety about how to talk about my surgeries when I got to university had been a waste. Now everyone knew. And more importantly, no one cared. Something occurred to me: it was only an issue if I made it into one.

The night went on. The dares continued. Everyone ran out of the room at one point to see one of the boys run around the quad naked – a dare – leaving me alone in The Boardroom with a very attractive boy, a friend of Alex's, who wasn't actually a resident of our block.

'I can't be bothered to go and watch,' I explained, standing to leave. 'I'm too tired. Actually, I think I'm going to go to bed – it's been a long night.'

'Oh, OK,' the boy said. 'If you're going to bed, I'll go and find everyone else.'

He followed me out of the room as I left. 'Well it was nice to meet you – good night,' I said.

That's when he put his hand on my cheek and started to kiss me. There is no exaggerating how surprised I was. The first boy I'd kissed hadn't known a thing about my scars. But this guy did. He had even seen them. *And he was still interested in me?*

We continued to kiss, and eventually found ourselves in the hallway near my room. 'Do I have to ask?' he said.

I hurriedly replied, 'No, of course not!' But I have to confess that I wasn't really sure what he meant. *Ask what?*

'Great.' He smiled, and grabbed my hand. 'Which way?' pointing down the corridor.

*Oh! That.*

'Wait,' I said. 'There's something you need to know. I've never done this before.'

He looked at me blankly. 'Don't worry, nor have I.'

As we arrived at the door to my room, I began to wonder whether he meant that he'd never had a one-night stand before – or whether he was a virgin like me.

'No,' I clarified. 'I mean I haven't done *any of this* before.'

'Oh!' he seemed surprised. 'Are you sure you want to?'

'Yes,' I said, 'but maybe not everything.'

Inside my room, he ran his hand across my scars. It was something I'd never imagined happening – to have them acknowledged in that way, and accepted.

'You know what,' I said after a while, 'let's try everything.'

In the cramped single bed, afterwards, his outstretched body took over the entire mattress. I had to grab hold of the bedside table to keep myself from falling out. As I clung to the table and tried to stay on the bed, my mind raced. *I barely spoke to him. We had one conversation at most. He's going to think I'm such a slut.* I worried that I was going to regret this in the morning.

Morning came and, rather than regret, I felt a great sense of excitement and relief. For years I had thought that any boy who saw my scars would bolt in disgust. The best I could hope for, I thought, was one day finding a man who would love me for my personality, enough to forgive me for my body. But I had been wrong. My one-night stand hadn't been attracted to my personality. He hadn't slept with me because I was funny or sarcastic or gregarious. He'd just wanted my body. Some might say he used me. I couldn't have been happier. It meant my body was worth using.

# 23

## What does it mean to be a woman?

One of the biggest revelations at university was that St Keyes had actually taught me some useful things – namely social skills. I arrived in Bristol with the ability to talk to virtually anyone and could start conversations easily. This skill had been honed over years of dull committee meetings, where I had to talk to parents and faculty alike, and at those terrible socials where I had suffered endless rejections. The upside: I could hide any social awkwardness and just plough on with a smile.

Most incredibly, this skill also applied to boys, despite my complete lack of experience with them. And now that I had stripped in front of my entire corridor, been kissed by Whatever-his-name-was from M Block, and even had sex, this new aspect of my social boldness was revealed.

At bars, clubs and parties, with alcohol to smooth the way, I soon realized that talking to boys was no different to talking to my friends. Boys were just as easy to talk to and I didn't even mind making the first move and starting the conversation.

The girls in my corridor marvelled at this. Before long, they were coming to me for advice about any number of sensitive subjects – tampons, periods, blowjobs, the pill, and whatever else I had picked up over the years in the St Keyes hothouse. After years of communal living at boarding school, I was comfortable with late-night confessional discussions – what we used to call 'DMCs', or deep-and-meaningful conversations. The nature of our chats at St Keyes had always been unfiltered – we didn't shyly ask for a tampon from a friend; we would announce it across the class – even if there was a male teacher. We didn't use weird pseudonyms when talking about sex; we called it what it was – penis, vagina, handjob, blowjob, sex. It wasn't until I was in the mixed halls of Bristol that I realized how controversial this was. I suddenly saw that my open demeanour earned me instant likeability and resulted in many of the girls on our floor confiding in me.

'I've known some of my friends back home all my life,' Chloe said one night, 'and we've never had conversations like this! I'd never even *said* the word blowjob before I met you.'

The opportunity to build a new reputation as being socially advanced – and wise – emboldened me further. I began approaching guys with a carefree attitude and an impenetrable wall of confidence. Being rejected by a guy no longer seemed a viable reason to stop putting myself out there. Unlike at a St Keyes social, if someone was rude, all I had to do was turn around and there would be another potential suitor.

As I advised my new friends, it was pointless to get side-tracked by insecurities – someone was always going to be rude, and that wasn't a reflection of us but of them. By going up to a boy at a bar, you had accomplished the hardest part and instantly made yourself the convenient choice. At St Keyes, we were taught that if you don't go after what you want, then you're never going to get it – and why was this any different? Why were we waiting for men to make their selection between us, when we could make our own decisions? I hated the idea of being compared to my friends and letting guys pick between us all. Approaching them saved me from that.

Before long, being typical freshers, we got into the habit of going out to local clubs every weekday evening and meeting boys, or just to dance with each other. On weekends, when clubs would fill with locals rather than students, we stayed on our corridor and played long games of Monopoly or card games in The Boardroom with containers of take-away food stacked around us. It was heaven.

In our common room there was a chart with two columns: a 'pull' column and a 'sex' column. Everybody's name was listed and had tallies next to it – of how many times. After a night out, the chart was updated and recalculated, with the person in question often refusing to admit exactly what they had done – because, unlike St Keyes, nobody wanted to have all the details of their sexual experiences tracked publicly – but their numbers escalated anyway.

There was still only one mark in my 'sex' column, but my 'pull' number was growing rapidly, due to my new-found skills. I was making up for lost time with long make-out sessions on the back wall of the Lizard Lounge and other clubs, after which a new number was calculated by my name. Sometimes I kissed several boys a night, or more. Only a few of these kisses had led to the exchanging of numbers, and certainly nothing close to a date, but that's how it was for almost all of us. Kissing and groping in the dark was like drinking and dancing – something to be done for fun, not a way to find a relationship. The exchange of numbers was mostly for texting about when we all planned to be at the Lizard Lounge again.

The girls in our corridor had concocted two rules that we deemed necessary to avoid being slut-shamed while living with so many boys, and kissing so many of them – and having the tally put up each morning on the common room chart.

1) No sex. You can do everything but. This would limit your 'number' from growing unnecessarily.
2) As long as you know his name, his course and his hall, you aren't a slut.

At the time, we didn't realize how ingrained 'lad culture' was even in our own beliefs; we didn't even recognize the vital flaws in this misogynistic system. We accepted it – of course, women are judged on their sexual acts. That's normal, isn't it? Isn't it normal to judge the girl who gives a blowjob at the cash machine but not the boy who receives it? Isn't it normal for him to be recognized with accolades and praise, while she's entrenched in shame for being so 'easy'? These double standards went unnoticed, and in our minds these precautions – these two rules – would keep us safe from the judgements of the world. Little did we know that this was just the start of a set of rules we would have to obey our entire lives in order to fit in with society's narrow view of what a woman should be.

As for the academic side of things, there wasn't too much pressure during that first year. At Bristol, your grades for the first year didn't count towards your actual degree; you just needed to pass and in doing so, you would start the second year off with a clean slate academically. Which meant that the first year – and in particular the first term – largely consisted of being drunk and hungover, with a notable lack of attendance at lectures. I found it harder and harder to get out of bed, and started waking later and later – and would only get up if a friend pounded on my door to invite me to lunch. After a few months of university life, I couldn't remember ever being so tired and sleepy, and put it down to a brutal combination of hangovers and freshers' flu. I began looking forward to spending the Christmas holidays at home in Hong Kong, so I could recover.

But once I got home, I was still sleeping fifteen hours a day and suffering from a terrible cold. I found it difficult to breathe and my snoring was so loud it could be heard throughout the house at night. My family began to complain. Sitting in the doctor's office, it was explained to me that I had glandular fever.

I was told this would mean no drinking and no kissing for the next four months – a pretty cruel predicament for a fresher. A choice would have to be made: I either had to stop going out entirely, which meant I'd miss out on all the fun times with my friends, or I could keep going out but remain sober. So, sober it was. I had some reservations around being able to keep up the overly sociable act without the aid of alcohol, but it had to be done. I had no choice – it was either that or risk losing my friends.

I returned to Bristol and continued my social pace as if nothing had happened – and to my surprise, very few people noticed the difference between my sober self and my drunk self anyway. Even without the hangovers, though, I had to sleep through the day to restore myself, and continued to miss classes. For the first time, I was able to make a choice about what to sacrifice due to illness, and it wasn't going to be my social life. I also found a new role to play: as I wasn't allowed to kiss anyone myself, I became the best wingwoman in the world, and enjoyed brazenly pushing my friends into guys in clubs, and making introductions.

On the occasional night that we didn't go out, I hung out with the boys in the common room or in one of their rooms. I learned so much. Their directness and honesty with each other was such a stark contrast to my previous experience of an all-girls atmosphere. But as I became an increasingly familiar presence in the common room, they became even less guarded and descended into crude discussions of other girls, sometimes describing them like objects: 'fit' or 'not fit', whether they were 'fuckable' or not. The lack of humanity was clear.

After a few times of hearing the term 'not fit', I voiced my annoyance. 'Some day, one of these girls is going to find out that you've said this and it's going to haunt her, and you will not only scar her for that evening, but for life,' I said. 'This is why people are self-conscious and how insecurities are born.'

Attempting to be sensitive and considerate, they immediately altered the phrase to 'not physically attractive' and began using that instead. It didn't make it any better, but I liked that they were trying at least. Despite all the roughness and bragging, they cared about what I thought.

Being dismissed as 'not fit' wasn't the worst assessment for a girl, though. I had overheard boys from other corridors talking in the dining hall about 'bagging', 'double-bagging' and 'triple-bagging'. The expression was used to describe a girl whose face they considered so ugly that it needed to be covered with a paper bag while they had sex. If they considered both her face and her body ugly, two bags were needed. The third expression was used if they thought the girl so ugly that they wouldn't even want their dog to see her. (In this case, they'd need a bag for the dog too.)

This was all dismissed as 'boy chat' – a phrase that not

only normalized it but undermined how truly appalling it was. As time passed, and we all became closer, these conversations grew less and less filtered. One time, a boy callously described a girl who was standing nearby as having 'legs like tree trunks', which made her run out of the room, while the rest of the girls eviscerated him.

'You don't know what kind of tree I was talking about!' the boy defended himself. 'Maybe I was talking about a thin tree with a spindly trunk.'

'You know very well what the phrase means,' a girl called out. 'And you know how any girl would take it!'

At St Keyes, bitching was our method of bonding and gossip was a currency, but upon arrival at Bristol I quickly learned that it wasn't the same here. Among the girls in V Block, bitching was not tolerated. If you bitched, the other girls would call you out on it, effectively stopping the conversation before it escalated. Boys didn't do that. Cruel comments were customary and often the others would join in as a competition in bravado, caving in to the peer pressure and wanting to keep up with this warped idea of masculinity. I'd seen it happen one night as we played a game of Truth or Dare. Alex was asked to choose who was best out of the two girls in the corridor he'd slept with. The room had exploded in laughter, and waited for his response.

'Don't you dare answer that!' I cried out before he was able to say anything. 'That question isn't funny.' I glared him down, repeating my warning over and over, while the crowd egged him on. Alex quietly blurted one girl's name. A low moment for him. I quickly looked around the room for the girl he hadn't chosen, but she'd gone. The damage had been done.

I had a rule of never sleeping with a boy from V Block – which meant I was never going to be the girl in a Truth or Dare question like that. Girls, in general, were measured on physical appearance and sexual ability far more than boys were. And when they ridiculed the opposite sex, the boys were clearly rougher and more wounding – even boys I liked and admired, whom I considered friends, and who would rip someone to shreds if they heard them talk about me like that. Yet they would do the same when talking about another girl. There seemed to be a different standard for the girls they saw as friends, from the ones they kissed or dated. This made me self-conscious. I couldn't help but imagine another corridor of boys having a similar conversation about me behind closed doors. I certainly lacked experience, so there was no chance that my sexual talents would rank very high. And I was hardly the 'perfect girl with the perfect body', the kind so often praised and honoured during these brutally honest drinking games.

One night, when I was talking to a room of girls, and feeling a bit vulnerable, I said: 'If you're a boy and can sleep with any other girl who has a normal body, why would you want to have sex with a girl who has a body like mine? I mean, it's like you're shopping and you want to buy a handbag. If you had a selection of handbags, you would never choose the one with scratches all over it, would you?'

A boy named George walked into the room just as I was saying that. He was a larger-than-life character – a big, loud, red-haired BNOC (Big Name on Campus) who was known for his extroverted personality. George was the kind of guy who climbed onto the table and burst into song midway through dinner – or just as easily came out with a string of offensive comments and somehow commanded the room. An honorary member of V Block, George was the captain of the football team and had the unexpected characteristic of being a devout Christian who didn't believe in sex before marriage. He was confident and vocal on this subject, openly defending it.

My first impressions of George hadn't been positive. The first time I met him I was sitting in the corridor with a friend, both of us minding our business, when out of nowhere he'd appeared in his football kit, in preparation for an upcoming game. As he passed us in the hallway, he spat in his gloves and smeared it on my face. I didn't even know his name. We'd truly never met. The next time I saw him, he started throwing squash balls at me. Once again, I'd been minding my business and simply talking to Alex in his room. The squash balls began flying around me – George clearly aiming for me. While I was really annoyed, I didn't want to give him my attention, so I ignored him.

Alex found my ability to do this amusing. 'Doesn't that hurt?' he asked.

'I don't care,' I replied, loudly enough so George could hear. 'Just as long as he doesn't hit my head.'

The next minute, George pelted my forehead with another ball. That did it. The expletives exploded from me and I explained that I'd had a number of surgeries on my head, that I had a tube in my neck that could break and send me back into the hospital again. Then I dissolved in tears. Shocked, George became apologetic. But it didn't stop him from always pushing the limits and seeing if he could provoke me, almost every time he saw me. One of his favourite jabs was chanting 'girl chat' whenever I tried to speak. It was all done in jest, but in my eyes, he crossed the line more often than not.

That day I compared my body to a damaged handbag, I could see he was gearing up to start his habitual banter as soon as he entered the room.

'*Wheyyy* Michelle,' he started in.

'Don't fuck with me, not today, George.'

Instead of coming up with some witty remark like he normally did, he simply said, 'OK,' and walked out. This kind of acquiescence on his part was unprecedented. The girls in the room looked at each other, puzzled.

'How did you do that?' one girl asked.

'He never leaves me alone when I ask him to,' another girl added.

I had no clue why he had respected my wishes. Then a few weeks later, on the last night of the Easter term, when everyone had gone out, I was roaming the corridor and looking for anybody as bored and sober as I was to talk to. I stumbled across George. He was sitting in Alex's room, typing at a keyboard.

'What are you doing?' I asked him. 'Does Alex know you're here?'

'Yes, he's letting me use his computer to finish off this essay. It's killing me.'

We started chatting and, for the first time, we had an actual decent conversation. No derision or abuse – probably because there was no audience for George to play to. After a few minutes, we decided to take a walk down to the local takeaway for dinner.

'By the way,' George said, as we were walking, 'a few weeks ago, when I walked in on you talking about a damaged handbag? You weren't talking about yourself, were you?'

'Yeah, I was,' I answered, embarrassed. 'I was just having a bad day.'

'Do you realize how ridiculous that is?' he said. 'I'm ginger. I have an afro. And I have psoriasis on my legs. I still have girls interested in me. What do you have to complain about?'

'You don't understand.' I paused, trying to decide how much to say. 'I have scars on my stomach and on my head and here and here and here,' I said, gesturing all over my body.

'I don't give a shit,' he said. 'You're a quality human and that's all that counts. Any arsehole that's going to walk away because of a few scars isn't worth your time.'

'I know, it's just—'

'Look at it this way,' he interrupted. 'Your scars are just a filtering process for all the douchebags in the world.

You're lucky. Most girls don't have that and they have to find out the hard way, months down the line.'

I thanked him, then grew silent for a moment, thinking about the wisdom of his remarks – and how good they made me feel.

'I know, I give bare good advice,' he said heartily – and just like that, his cocky arrogant self was back.

Perhaps we all have things to hide, I thought. Things we don't like about ourselves, things we know aren't perfect. We can focus on them and obsess over them, but the obsession doesn't stop the insecurities existing. I would never have guessed that George was insecure – I had no clue about his psoriasis and all the aspects that he thought made him stereotypically unattractive – being ginger, having an afro. I'd never thought twice about it. Was all this 'lad chat' just a way to deflect from their own insecurities? Perhaps there was truth in what he was saying. Perhaps if he thought like that, other boys might too? I wasn't sure how I'd ever come to love my scars, but perhaps the trick was just to act like I did. The blasé, natural way in which George had described his imperfections as simple facts, without judgement – I needed that.

As the weather grew warmer, the girls on our corridor decided to participate in a 5k charity run for breast cancer. Wanting to be part of the team, I signed up, knowing that I would have to train. To be honest, just the thought of running any distance brought up a wealth of bad sporting memories from school, particularly my failures in cross-country. Over lunch, after I'd shared my St Keyes memories, Freddie piped up.

'I'll help you!' he said. 'I want to improve my running anyway.' While it was a lovely offer, the thought of exercising in front of Freddie wasn't appealing. He was easily the sportiest boy in our corridor and the idea of huffing and panting in front of him – out of breath and exhausted – was completely embarrassing. I thanked him for the offer, secretly hoping he would swiftly forget about it.

The following day, he knocked on my door. 'Let's go for a run!' he said excitedly.

'Freddie, this is silly,' I said, backing away. 'Just to stay with me, you'll have to run so slowly it'll be boring for you.'

'We're going to do suicides,' he said, insisting, 'so we'll stay in the same area. I've come up with a whole plan. It'll be like boot camp. Come on! You have a 5k to run. You have to train!'

'Suicides' are a way of training in short blasts at top speed, between trees. Freddie walked me to his planned area for our boot camp, which turned out to be right in front of all the halls and where everyone on the bus could watch as they went past.

'I'm doing twenty, you do fifteen,' he said. 'It's a race – come on, between these two trees, go!'

Before long I had forgotten about the people on the bus or what I might look like sweating in front of Freddie. I lost myself in the gruelling exercise and the competitiveness.

It turned out that the competitiveness from St Keyes was still alive in me somewhere.

'I have one last exercise,' he said. 'Here – hold my hand!'

I grabbed a hold of his hand, clasping tightly. As soon as I did, he began running. 'Come on, keep up!' he cried out. 'Keep holding my hand!' His legs picked up speed. Soon he was sprinting.

'Freddie, slow down! I'm going to fall…'

He continued to sprint, his sweaty palm keeping a tight grip over mine. I started to understand the rush people felt when they exercised. It was liberating, exhilarating – and for the first time, I felt a sense of freedom that I hadn't ever felt before. Even more so, for the first time, exercise had led to a connection to my body that seemed over and beyond its appearance. Unlike at St Keyes, exercise now seemed a personal accomplishment rather than an excuse for comparison. I didn't need to be good at it – I just had to enjoy it. These workouts continued a couple times a week, and on the way back to the hall we would often bump into Freddie's friends. I had to meet them while sweat-covered and makeup free and I got used to that. Over the years at St Keyes, being makeup free had been my norm, but since then I'd felt pressure to conform to all these beauty standards – especially in the presence of guys. To be free of that pressure on these encounters was liberating and felt more natural, even comforting.

Before long, I started to have confidence in my sporting ability and alongside it, a new and unlikely friendship.

A week before the 5k event, Freddie was unable to make our usual session, so I encouraged Chloe to come instead. She was also running in the race, but hadn't prepared. She and I proceeded to the area where Freddie and I had our boot camps. Midway through our circuits, I began to notice the difference between exercising with a muscular, tall, built man like Freddie and training with Chloe.

Each car that passed us honked or yelled abuse out the window.

'Run, fatty, run!'

Chloe became upset and asked to go back inside, but I was spurred on. 'They're a bunch of strangers. Why should we care what they think?' I cried out through gulps of air. Perhaps it was something I'd learned in the hospital, or the lasting effects of St Keyes, but suddenly, in that moment, all my energy went into proving them wrong. I refused to let some stranger detract from my enjoyment. My body was about more than what it looked like – and I pitied those strangers for not being able to see that.


At the end of my first year at Bristol, I booked an appointment at the tattoo parlour. In less than a year, I had gone from not being able to talk about my surgeries to finally accepting my past as a part of me. My surgeries, my scars and my illness were no longer a secret and I wanted to commemorate that. I had the fantastic idea of putting the number thirteen permanently on my foot – a skin symbol of the fact that I had nothing to hide any more.

Every single person on the corridor tried to dissuade me. 'You're doing *what*?'

'Are you kidding?'

'What's the rush?'

'Just think about it more.'

'Don't do something you'll regret.'

I had always been proud but also superstitious about being born on Friday the thirteenth, believing it could explain why bad luck had followed me throughout my life. This was my way of reclaiming my power. And the placement of the tattoo on my foot was how I would be reminded that my past would impact each step I took. I never wanted to go back to hiding parts of myself or carrying my own history as baggage. This tattoo was going to be my way of guaranteeing that.

'Do you even know what you want the tattoo to look like?' one of my friends asked.

No, I had no clue. So we sat down at a computer and scrolled through various fonts in Word, selecting one and then, with a regular pen, copying it onto my foot. When I walked around with '13' written on my bare foot, all my friends laughed. They were sure that I wasn't going to follow through.

Twenty-four hours later, though, it was there – a real tattoo stamped permanently on my skin, and in a very visible and prominent position. Proudly, I posted a photograph of it on my Facebook wall. This prompted rumours among my St Keyes circle that I had changed and 'gone rebellious'. Girls from St Keyes didn't get tattoos. This made my new mark even more satisfying; it meant I no longer fit into their narrow stereotype of who I was or how I should behave – that neat box that made me a St Keyes production.

Years ago, my scars were created by someone else. But now I had marked myself. This body alteration was one I could control. And the number itself was a declaration that I refused to carry my thirteen surgeries as a secret inside of me and instead, would be proudly declared on my skin. That summer, after a trip to Japan, I would get another one to add to my collection. This time, one on my wrist of a bow that was made out of closed circles.

My tattoos weren't just my talismans; they made my body mine again. I had reclaimed my body, my way.

# 24

## What is love?

My second year at Bristol brought a boy into my life. I was at my favourite club, the Lizard Lounge – a place known for cheesy music and sticky floors, but to most of V Block, it was bliss. Despite no longer living in the same block, we were all still friends but because we had all split into three separate houses, the Lizard Lounge remained our meeting point. We went every Thursday and proudly announced how much we loved it, while the rest of the university seemed ashamed to be there.

I saw Alex standing by the bar with a friend. I walked up to talk to them, interrupting their conversation midway before realizing what I'd done – and that I hadn't introduced myself. Alex's friend, a tall, broad-shouldered guy with the cheekiest smile, told me his name was Luke. Then he asked what degree I was doing. Always the first question.

'Ugh. Psychology,' he said. 'Can you read my mind?'

I couldn't help but roll my eyes. I'd heard this comment so many times that fighting the stereotype had become boring. 'Yes, but trust me, you don't want me to say what you're thinking out loud,' I replied with a grin. 'Anyway, what do you do?'

'Computer science,' he said, hesitating, as if embarrassed.

'And you were judging *me*? You must have to deal with worse stereotypes than I do.'

'Sorry,' he went on. 'It's just that my mother is a social worker so I know your type and I don't really want to be psychoanalysed tonight.'

'Wow. Now you're comparing me to your *mother*? Don't worry, I know computer scientists aren't known for their social skills so I'll let you off the hook.'

He laughed and offered to buy me a drink. Guys never did that unless we'd spent the night kissing or something. And rather than kissing, Luke only pecked me on the cheek a few times while we talked for hours. When he mouthed the words to 'Hottest Girl in the World' in a goofy but adorable way, I was charmed. At the end of the night, he asked for my number, but didn't push things to go any further – something I noticed because it was so far from the norm.

The following morning I went to my lecture, still dazed from the night before. I sat down and my phone buzzed.

Hope your 9 am wasn't too painful x

*Aw how sweet*, I thought. A huge smile beamed across

my face. He had even remembered what time my lecture was – so much more romantic than any other boys I knew.

Luke and I continued texting every day for the next week. Then a little dance began. If he waited three hours before replying, then I would wait four hours. After that, he would wait five hours to text me again, then I would wait five-and-a-half. Then, excited by the delay, one kiss – 'X' – got pushed up to two.

There was no mention of a date, but I expected to see him on Thursday at the Lizard Lounge. However, Thursday came and went with no sign of him in the club. Even worse, he hadn't replied to me for twenty-four hours. I was starting to worry that it was over. I guessed I'd blown it somehow.

The following evening, I was invited to three house parties – a normal occurrence for a university night – and at the last one, I entered a bustling room filled with fifty people and noticed Luke standing in the corner looking at his phone. This really annoyed me. 'Look! He's texting!' I vented to Emma. 'But he couldn't be bothered to reply to my last text?'

Just as I spoke those words, my phone pinged and I looked down to see his reply. Laughing, I walked over to him, phone in hand. 'Hi there!'

He looked up from his phone with a mixture of confusion, shock and embarrassment that I had caught him standing alone in the corner of a house party, texting.

'What are you doing here?'

As soon as we began to talk, somehow all the other

people in the room became invisible. Time flew and before I knew it, my housemates were heading home. 'You coming with us?' one of them asked. 'Or are you staying?'

If I stayed, I knew Luke would walk me home and most likely, he would stay over. A part of me wanted this more than anything, but an old inner nightmare began playing in my head: how was I going to tell him about my scars? I went back and forth, changing my mind about whether to leave or stay, until it was decided for me as my house-mates had already left. We talked and kissed. Then he offered to walk me home.

My friends had all reassured me that boys didn't need a 'warning' about my body. But as Luke and I walked, I tried to imagine ways to say it, ways to break the news that would soften the surprise. For years I had lived with a fear that I'd be alone with a boy, pull off my top, and he'd run from the room in horror. Despite having experienced the opposite in the first year, it was still a major insecurity. This also seemed like more of a risk since I cared more about Luke's opinion more than all the previous guys. If Luke looked at me with disgust, it would destroy me. I started looking for any chance to tell him, to warn him, before that happened.

Distracted by my thoughts, I tripped while walking down the hill. 'Whoops, sorry! I'm so clumsy!' I laughed as I grabbed onto him, and kept myself from falling.

'You can't be as clumsy as my brother,' Luke said in a reassuring voice. 'He has dyspraxia!' He wrapped his arm around me and pulled me closer.

'So do I, actually, and dyslexia too,' I blurted out – suddenly seeing my chance to raise other medical matters. 'And I've also kind-of had a brain tumour, and then I have this thing called hydrocephalus and messed-up intestines and all kinds of things. I've had, like, thirteen other operations too.'

I was jabbering like a panicked schoolgirl. But in my drunken haze, I believed that I had brilliantly mastered a transition between two tangentially related conversation topics. Luke gave no direct response to this onslaught of information. As we continued to walk, it dawned on me that I had given him a laundry list of my medical conditions – from A to Z in under twenty seconds – but no mention of scars. It was too late. We were already talking about something completely different.

So, once in my bedroom, before removing any clothing, I raised it again. 'You know those surgeries?'

He was kissing me, and interrupting each word I spoke. 'Hmmm?'

'They left me with scars, by the way—'

'*Shhhhh*,' he whispered through kisses.

I hesitated before removing any clothes. 'You ready?' I asked. Then I pulled my top over my head and completely missed the reaction on his face. By the time I could see it, he was looking down at me – just staring at the scars and saying nothing. Then he placed his hand on them and continued kissing me on the cheek.

'They're beautiful,' he said. 'I don't know what you were so worried about.'

*

Luke and I met at the Lizard Lounge most Thursdays after that. We'd text, and see each other across the bar. Sometimes we'd be flirting with other people, or just talking with friends. But when the evening was drawing to a close, he would always come to find me, kiss me. One time, he blurted out the words 'I love you' and I responded with a laugh – the idea seemed utterly ludicrous to me – which led him to retracting it and replacing it with 'I mean, I really, really like you'. But that night, and on a number that followed, we kissed, shared a conversation, then went our separate ways. Weeks passed and we still hadn't been on a proper date. I began to wonder if we ever would.

On the final night of term, before Christmas break, when we were standing outside the Lizard Lounge and kissing, he blurted it out again: 'I love you.'

I didn't laugh this time. And he made no attempt to retract it. By then, we'd known each other for three months. And while I didn't say it back to him – the words would have stuck in my throat – we did go home together. Whatever was happening with Luke, we were moving in the right direction. Our inevitable first date would come after the Christmas holidays, right?

# 25

## Is anything simple?

It was almost fated that as soon as I got the tattoo to ward off further trips to the hospital, I would end up there. And sure enough, my holiday plans at home in Hong Kong included a medical procedure. Glandular fever had persisted – preventing me from sleeping properly and even breathing well at times. It was decided that I needed to have my tonsils and adenoids removed.

How rough could this simple surgery be? My brother had had the procedure when he was seven with no dramas. If he could do it, so could I. Because of how the term dates worked out, I would have the surgery on the day before New Year's Eve, 2012 – and recover afterwards. That was a relief. At least the operation would happen before 2013 started. Ever since that St Keyes girl had joked that I would die in 2013, this fear had stayed with me.

And things went well, initially. Less than a week after

the procedure, I was back on my feet, fully recovered. Even better, Luke was finally texting me properly. He hadn't texted me much since the Christmas holidays began and while I worried that it may be a bad sign, I also knew that he was on a university ski trip with all my closest friends, was most likely busy, and occasionally would send a picture or a joke, or say that he missed me. By this time, I missed him desperately and was excitedly packing and preparing to return to university.

Just before leaving, I made plans to see my old friend Marissa, whom I'd known since primary school. In Hong Kong, nights out start very late and it's customary to stay out until dawn. It was almost eleven o'clock and I was still at home, getting ready in my room, when I felt a dull kick to my stomach. The pain came and went suddenly. I didn't think much more about it.

I went downstairs for a bite of food and felt another kick – a dull burst of pain.

'Ouch!'

'What is it?' my dad asked.

'Nothing,' I said. 'My stomach is starting to hurt. I think I might have eaten something funny.'

'Well, don't go out then.'

'It's too late to cancel,' I replied. 'Marissa has already left the house. I'll drink some water and I'm sure I'll be fine.'

On the taxi ride to Lan Kwai Fung, the nightclub district of Hong Kong, I felt another burst of pain, then it disappeared for five minutes. By the time I met Marissa, the pain had become more frequent – and grown sharper. I told myself it was just food poisoning. And maybe some alcohol would ease the pain. Saying nothing to Marissa, I just tried to enjoy the night. But the pain grew sharper and sharper. An hour later, I finally said something.

'I keep getting this pain in my stomach! These short, sharp stabs – at first they were five minutes apart but now the intervals are less than a minute.'

Marissa laughed. 'Could you be pregnant?' she asked. 'You've just described contractions! When was the last time that you had sex?'

Luke. Our last night together had been three weeks before. The first time we'd gotten together had been only two months before that... The timing didn't add up, but my mind swirled and made connections and associations. Episodes of the TV show *I Didn't Know I Was Pregnant* started running through my head. In one storyline, the woman becomes improbably pregnant not from sex, but during foreplay.

No. That's absurd. Food poisoning. It has to be food poisoning.

But an hour later, I could barely stand. Buckled over, clutching my stomach, I finally admitted defeat and went home, where I proceeded to drink two litres of water, believing this would 'flush' whatever bug was in my system. Then I curled into a ball on my bed and tried to sleep. An hour later, going back and forth to the bathroom, nothing had changed.

My brother, noticing that my light was on, came in.

'What's wrong? Did you get too drunk?' A few minutes later, my mum appeared. 'What's the matter? Why are you home so early? Why are you lying in bed with the light on?' They were both talking about the hospital – and thought that I needed to go.

'I think I have food poisoning,' I muttered. 'I don't know.'

My mum started running through what I had eaten that day, trying to determine what had made me sick. Only half an hour later, when the pain wasn't any better, I conceded.

'Fine, I'll go to hospital,' I said. 'If only to prove to you that I'm fine. You are both so dramatic!'

At the hospital, I began apologizing for wasting the doctor's time. I was sure it was just food poisoning. And much to my relief, he agreed with me. 'I'm pretty sure you're right,' he said. 'You probably have nothing to worry about.'

'See, I told you!' I said to Mum. Standing to open the door, I felt another pang of pain and before I knew it, I had covered the walls of the room with my dinner, and continued to projectile vomit for the next few minutes. The doctor suggested that I spend the night in hospital. He still believed it was probably food poisoning, but there was a chance it could be something more serious.

He explained that earlier in the day he'd treated a patient who had experienced similar symptoms and it turned out to be an 'obstructed bowel'.

*Obstructed bowel?* What on earth was that? The doctor immediately reassured me that it was unlikely, but as a precaution, I would be linked up to a drip to feed me nutrients and give me some medication to help me sleep. I tried to mention that I'd had sex – and could be pregnant – but I didn't know how to say those things in front of my mum. A night in hospital wasn't the worst thing I'd been through. Now, with the drugs kicking in, I could finally sleep.

# 26

## Will I ever be normal?

My eyes slowly opened to see a hypodermic needle being inserted into my arm. I noticed my parents in the corner of my hospital room, having a conversation with a doctor I didn't recognize.

Earlier that morning, before being taken for X-rays and scans, I'd been asked a series of intrusive questions that are not usually asked in front of one's parents. The paranoia that I could be pregnant was still playing on my mind when the doctor began whispering to my parents. Then he came to my bedside. 'We know what's wrong,' he said. 'You're going to need an operation.'

Indeed, my bowel was obstructed. Most likely, it was a result of my abdominal surgery years before; the adhesions or scar tissue can cause lingering complications.

'It's only a small operation,' the doctor said, 'a small cut on your stomach.'

'I've heard that before.'

He tried to reassure me. 'Look,' he said, 'we can make the incision right on top of one of your previous scars, so you won't even see it. I did this procedure just yesterday, and the woman is already going home.'

'No... I'm not doing it,' I stated, defiantly.

As it turned out, I didn't have a choice.

I'd been supposed to fly back to England the following day. That wasn't going to happen. There'd be no happy return to Luke. And even worse, now that it was 2013, the prophecy of doom was coming about. There was nothing to do but burst into tears.


The loneliness of waking after surgery was familiar, but that didn't make it any easier to bear. Listening to the sounds of the monitors, and taking in the sights and smells of the hospital, I felt little again, weak, like a small thin girl of eleven who was far away from home and scared, alone and uncertain about what was going to happen next.

A week passed. I was doing well, the doctor said, and making a quick recovery. This gave me hope, and helped to drive away the memories of the past, when surgeries always seemed to be followed by more complications, and more surgeries. I was still in pain from the abdominal surgery, unable to sit up and still bed-ridden, but soon it was time to start eating again, and the nurses began easing me back onto solid food. They said I could eat whatever I wanted. Having gone for a week without food in my mouth, or in my stomach, I was ambitious. I ate and shortly afterwards, I began feeling sick. A few moments later, I was sick.

Not to worry, the nurses explained. This happened occasionally. They gave me more pain medication. I nodded off, and a couple of hours later I awoke in excruciating abdominal pain, and began to throw up again.

I reached for the call button, but it had fallen to the floor. I began yelling, hoping to be heard by a nurse in the corridor. I waited, but nobody came. In the children's ICU, I would have been heard. But in a regular adult ward, nurses were scarce. I cried, knowing that I wasn't supposed to cry – a strain on my fluid supply, hard on my abdominal muscles, and a dip in potassium. My only hope was the night-shift nurses, who would soon be making their rounds.

Two hours later, a nurse did enter my room to check one of my drips – and found me covered in my own vomit, which had dried all around me. One look at my tear-stained face told her the story. I remained awake for the rest of the night, just staring at the wall.

All I wanted was to be normal and healthy again – to be walking down the street, going to class, without a care in the world. How had I taken all that for granted? The ability to walk, the broad ranges of flavours that food brings, a glass of water, to go to the toilet unaccompanied, to laugh without a stabbing pain in my stomach... Simple things now seemed like luxuries.

After that night, my mum refused to leave me alone and slept on the sofa in my hospital room. She was trying to be helpful, thinking of my care and recovery, but it made things worse. Each night, I tried to be mindful of waking her, careful not to let her see the glare of my laptop screen. She kept telling me to put it away, to get some sleep. Without it, I watched Mum drift off and then continued to stare at the wall in front of me in hope that the pain would subside and the thoughts would disperse, allowing me to sleep.

A few days later, a new scan revealed that my bowel was obstructed again – but only partially. That was why I couldn't keep food down. This was disguised as good news. They focused on the fact that I wouldn't need a surgery and instead all I needed was time so that my intestines could untangle themselves on their own. The doctors tried to be encouraging, and I tried to believe them, but they'd been wrong too many times before. Days began to pass in a blur. I thought about Luke and checked my phone for texts from him, but none came. I listened to One Direction's new album. And I opened my laptop again. Locked away in a hospital room, immobile in bed, not able to eat food or drink water, I was beginning to accept that this might continue for weeks – and that it might result in another surgery.

By this time, I had stopped blaming Luke for not texting me. Why would he bother? When you enter a hospital you become invisible – a nonentity who may never get better, or even live. Somehow, over the years, I had convinced myself that I was normal and healthy and could have a normal life like other people, but now my whole future seemed unsupportable. At any moment, the foundation that I had built – all the friends and contacts I had accumulated – could crumble. There was no hope that I'd ever be normal. The most I could hope for, or probably deserved, was 'convenient love' – a love that would be there conditionally, until I went into hospital again. After all, if I were given the choice, I wouldn't choose this, so why would he?

It felt like beneath my hospital bed there was a gaping hole that had swallowed all the happiness that had been created, leaving devastation in its wake. These are the kinds of thoughts you have while you're not recovering successfully from your fifteenth surgery and your bowels are tied in knots.

# 27

## Will I ever go home?

On the rare days I was feeling better, Marissa would visit and attempt to cheer me up. Marissa had been my first best friend, and was the complete opposite of me. She was sporty and popular. Her visits made a world of difference. She brought me movies from our childhood to watch, music to keep me updated, and she aided my childish pranks, much to the nurses' annoyance.

Social media helped too. Years before, during my long hospital stay at UCLA when I was eleven, there had been no such comfort. Now, technology had entered all aspects of daily life and made my recovery bearable – almost enjoyable. Some days, my friends at university would leave their Skype open on their laptops, while I was on the other end, making me feel as if I was in the room. The university had given me an extension on all my deadlines, since I was still tethered to an IV drip and had difficulty typing or moving my hands. Sometimes I looked down at my black-and-blue battered wrists from the IV, noticed my tattoo and would try in vain to remember a time when I was happy. As time dragged on, Facebook became a less positive experience. It had started snowing in England and photos of my friends in the snow started appearing. With each day of missing out, I grew more fearful that I would be forgotten, the way I had been at St Keyes.

It was on one of these mornings, when I was feeling forlorn, that I began to take umbrage at the way my Facebook friends expressed themselves online. Their choice of words and phrases – things like 'could this day get any worse?' and 'I'm going to die if I have another deadline' or 'I'm going to kill myself if I don't finish this essay' – began to infuriate me. So I decided to block all social media on my phone and laptop, and delete my accounts. It was pointless to post depressing updates about my day; they would only make my friends feel guilty, pity me or prompt them to say they wished I was there – the kind of thing everybody says to someone who's missing out on fun. My endless online stalking was only making things harder; it started to make me want to lash out about how unaware these people were of the privileges of being healthy. Rather than risking losing all my friends, I just turned off my phone, absorbed myself in the latest TV shows, and went into a deep depression.

Just when I was hitting a total low, my mum and god-mother, Evangeline, arrived and took over a corner of my room. Evangeline – my mum's best friend – was the epitome of glamour, with perfectly coiffed blonde hair and stylish clothes. The two of them were locked in a conversation about their wrinkles and sagging skin, complaining that they had jowls and crow's feet. They touched their lovely faces, lifting their cheeks and eyelids with their fingers while they talked about how terrible they looked.

Wrinkles made a person seem more beautiful to me. When I saw crow's feet around someone's eyes, I thought of all the laughing they must have done in life, how many moments lived and enjoyed.

'Please change the subject,' I said.

They looked at me, puzzled.

'I don't want to hear any more about your wrinkles.'

'You're too young to understand!' they cried out in unison. This was followed by a string of defensive comments. They made getting older and having a few wrinkles sound like the world was coming to an end.

'Ageing is a privilege!' I cried out.

This statement was met with more confusion. Both my mum and Evangeline were shaking their heads. 'Ageing isn't a privilege!' my mum replied. 'It happens to all of us.'

'Yes,' I responded. 'It happens to people *who live*. Would you prefer the alternative? Anti-ageing literally means dying.'

The previous day, I had seen a video on YouTube in which a collection of people who were dying described their regrets. It was very powerful, but I couldn't help but notice that everybody in the video was over eighty. They had lived a long time, presumably a full life, and were now focusing on all the things they hadn't got to do. This enraged me. But where were the dying children? Not everyone gets the chance to live until they're eighty.

Every day there was a battle. Every day there was something new that enraged me. My parents would nag me to have a shower or brush my hair but frankly, I saw no point. People kept saying it would 'make you feel better', but I liked looking exactly as bad as I felt.

My mum said that I was starting to smell. But getting in the shower was a painful process, and required me to sit in a position that pressed on my incision site while I tried to avoid getting any area of my stomach wet. Worst of all, my mum had to stand there and scrub me like a baby.

Control is underrated, and most of us don't give it enough thought. But until you lose it, you aren't really aware of how much it matters. Being in the hospital felt like being in prison, except in prison, you know how long your sentence is and meals come regularly. Instead, I envisaged being stuck there while my friends finished out the term, went on to graduate, got married and began having babies.

I started hiding under my duvet. Under the bedcovers, I could cry without being seen. I could finally have silence and be alone. When my parents came to visit, they were unable to convince me to surface. When my sister came, she got me to uncover my face long enough to say goodbye.

By then, my friends had become alarmed that I'd deleted my social media pages. They began texting.

Are you ok? What's happening?

They worried that I'd died. Replying to them, other than to reassure them that I was alive, became hard. As soon as I told them I was still in the hospital, and they said they were sorry, it seemed they couldn't wait to tell me about their latest boy dramas and friendship gossip and university crises. And that made me cry.

They cared. I know they did. But talking to them made my life harder, made me feel even more alone and isolated. The grim reality that it could be weeks or months before I could eat a regular meal, or feel the fresh air on my skin, or be back in England again and having fun with my friends, haunted me. When I did come out from under my duvet cover, there were only five words to say: *I want to go home.*

# 28

## Am I in control?

Worried about my mental state, the doctors held whispered conferences in the corridor outside my room. It was early in the morning when three of them walked in, accompanied by my parents. I was in my safe place, under the duvet.

'Michelle, you're going to want to hear this,' my dad said.

I didn't reply.

'Michelle, you're going home,' one of the doctors announced.

*Huh?* I slowly surfaced with a hesitant smile, wondering whether this was truth – or a ploy. 'What do you mean? I haven't been able to poo yet. And I'm not able to eat.'

'Well, you're right,' the doctor said, 'but since all you're doing here is waiting, you might as well be waiting at home. Your parents are going to fill out the paperwork to discharge you, and hopefully once you're home and more active, your body will take the hint and start working again.'

I crawled out of bed. Ecstatic, I began packing up my room. I was in bliss as my wheelchair rolled out of the hospital doors. Fresh air! Sounds of life – of car engines and birds chirping and people talking – that weren't heart monitors! My mum drove up to the front of the hospital and my dad helped me out of the chair, and into our car.

But the car was so high. I had never realized how high it was. With a noticeable absence of stomach muscles, climbing into the back seat was nearly impossible. It was a strain just to lift my leg high enough to begin the first step. I plastered a smile on my face, hoping that it would make my difficulty less noticeable and perhaps reduce the pain as I slowly edged and hoisted myself into the back seat. Eventually settled in, my dad closed the door and sat next to me as my mum set off. *I really didn't think this through.*

As the car drove along, I felt each turn of the wheel, each bump in the road. The tyres jostled and rumbled, and I felt it in my stomach, as though my incision were being pulled apart. Each turn of a corner threw my body off-kilter. I attempted to balance myself, while continuing to fake a smile, not wanting my parents to see what I was going through.

Finally at home, I spent the rest of the day with my dad watching TV in the living room. And that was nice. With the absence of nutrition from IV drips, I was not allowed to eat but was allowed an occasional sip of Gatorade to keep my electrolytes up. I took a shower alone and restored my hygiene levels and comforted myself with cosy thoughts of sleeping in my own bed for a change. But then I realized something important. In the hospital, the bed raised and lowered – and I didn't have to use my abdominal muscles to sit up. My bed at home didn't have a lift or motor. Once I was there, I was helpless. Whatever position I was in would remain my position, unless physically moved or rolled over by somebody else. I required assistance to even sit up.

I passed the evening lying down, and yelling for my mum every time I thought I might throw up, which was quite often, now that the Gatorade was hitting my stomach. So I shifted my position again, very slowly, and sat in a chair, where I was able to reach a sink if I needed to. I spent the night like that, in a chair, staring at a wall, hoping to fall asleep (but I couldn't) and constantly feeling that I wanted to throw up (but I couldn't). As the sun began to enter through the windows of my room, I finally drifted off.

A matter of minutes later, my mum walked in.

'Why are you sleeping in a chair?' she asked.

It was useless to argue. The experiment had been a failure from the beginning. My return to the hospital was immediate and unremarkable, except that it brought vague relief and gratitude. I would no longer need to overexert myself or pretend nothing was wrong. And I'd never realized how nice a hospital bed could be.

\*

There were more whispered conferences in the corridor, and meetings. Multiple scans later, and a change of doctors, the state of my bowels had still not changed. One morning, the doctors and my parents gathered in my room to tell me the next plan of action. They were going to insert a needle in my neck. I don't remember what the purpose of this needle was, and it really didn't matter. There was nothing more terrifying to me. My neck had always been very sensitive – I rarely let my friends touch it when they went to hug me.

Weeping and hysterical, I begged the doctors just to operate on the bowel obstruction instead. As a compromise, they agreed to delay the procedure for three days, in the hope that a few more enemas and suppositories might jumpstart my digestive system. If I wasn't able to poo within that time, the needle would go in my neck. And if that failed, there would be another surgery. My sweet sixteenth.

Ordinarily, I wasn't too wild about inserting my own fingers up my bum, and putting in a suppository, but if that meant avoiding a needle in my neck, so be it. These were doctor's orders. Glove on, the suppository was placed on my two forefingers, lubrication around it, and I would attempt to relax as I contorted myself to reach my own arsehole. They gave me the option to let the nurse do it, but that seemed worse. It was like a bad game of 'would you rather'.

*Would you rather only be able to drink your own piss for a week or drink a cup of your period blood?*

*Would you rather shove your own fingers up your bum or would you rather a nurse did it for you?*

Whether it was the threat of the needle in my neck, the threat of my sixteenth surgery, or the fact that both my best friends had birthdays quickly approaching, I don't know. But my recalcitrant intestines finally kicked into gear. Almost on cue, I had my first bowel movement.

My parents were proud. I was beaming. It was a picture-worthy celebration, much like your first poo in the potty. Except my friends weren't as grateful for the update.

# 29

## Skinny or healthy?

Food had not passed my lips for six weeks. Not even a drop of water. You'd think this would become normal after a while, but the primal human desire to smell, chew, taste and swallow real food doesn't go away. It becomes more intense.

Thoughts of food began to consume me and I spent days and nights in the hospital scrolling on Instagram through the hashtags #foodporn or #chocolate to try to even remember what it was like to have something sweet or savoury in my mouth. When I was finally allowed to walk, things only became worse. On my daily strolls for exercise, I would pass hospital rooms where lunches and dinners were being served. Somehow my sense of smell had become more acute, a kind of hyper-vigilant superpower that allowed me to detect exactly what was on a patient's plate many rooms away. And while walking, I followed the best smells and would linger at the doorway of a diner's room just to get a glimpse of a cheeseburger.

Occasionally, my laps around the hospital ward would coincide with meal trays being placed in the corridor for collection and I was taunted by the half-consumed dinners, the stray pile of cold French fries, smudges of ketchup, or even a lettuce leaf. One night, I was so desperate for food that I began bartering with one of the nurses for a mere grain of rice, after negotiating down from chocolate.

'Come on, rice is plain!' I begged her. 'I just *need something*. I need to feel the sensation of chewing. I promise that I won't press the call button for a whole hour, a whole day. I'll become the best patient ever.' But there was no way to convince her.

My dramatic weight loss, meanwhile, was prompting compliments from my nurses, parents, godparents and siblings. A steady stream of visitors to my room all said things like:

'You look fantastic!'

'You face looks skinnier.'

'You actually look good – much healthier without the extra weight.'

It frustrated me that weight loss was praised even in the context of illness. Was skinny still the goal if your health had to be at risk in order to achieve it?

When I'd entered the hospital, aged nineteen, I was coincidentally the slimmest and fittest I'd been in years. I'd stopped analysing and measuring what I was eating. I ate what I wanted, when I wanted and had the healthiest relationship with food I'd ever had before – not because I was eating the healthiest, but because my days no longer revolved around food. I'd also become more comfortable with my scars. My tattoos had signified a shift in my mentality around my body and the only thing that still bothered me was 'my number'. I weighed about 200 pounds (or 90 kg) – medically my BMI was morbidly obese, yet my dress size was a fourteen. It made no sense. Perhaps it had something to do with all the metal shunts and plastic tubing in my body, along with the copious amounts of scar tissue? But it was a number I still worried about.

Before I'd returned to Hong Kong, I'd been reminded of how big the number '200' seemed to most people, when I was with a group of friends from V Block. We were playing a game of cards when Freddie and Alex started discussing how they'd been bulking up. In passing, Freddie mentioned that he now weighed 200 pounds.

'We weigh the same, then,' I said, without thinking too much about it, continuing to shuffle the deck of cards.

'What – you weigh 200 pounds?' he said, clearly shocked.

I knew what he was thinking. Freddie was much taller than me, and built of pure muscle. How could we possibly weigh the same?

'You look much skinnier than you weigh!' he said, fumbling a bit. I'd heard this time and time again, so continued to shuffle the cards, unreactive.

The girls around our table interrupted in outrage. 'Freddie! *That's so rude!*' They each chimed in with more criticisms, saying how mean Freddie was. I hadn't registered it as a comment that was intended to insult. I knew he wasn't being mean, but being defended by all the girls at the table left me embarrassed that they thought he was. Were they thinking the same? Was that number as horrifying as the looks on their faces suggested?

When I ran out of the room crying, Freddie chased after me and explained that he was only surprised because I didn't look like I weighed as much as he did – and besides, he said, 'I have no idea how much anybody weighs.'

This incident lingered in my mind as I waited to leave the hospital. I knew that each day I didn't eat real food – and existed only on the necessary nutrients being fed to me by an IV drip – the more weight I would lose. And the more compliments I would get. But I felt like I should have been warning all my visitors, and myself, not to grow attached to this 'New Me', because it wouldn't last. There was no doubt. As soon as I left the hospital and began eating again, the pounds would start piling on, as they always did.

I would gain it all back – and then some. This happens after any extreme diet or extreme weight loss from illness: it's a proven physiological response. The sudden restriction of food sends your body into starvation mode, your metabolism slows way down and your body clings onto the fat as a way of protecting yourself. This causes your weight to climb at an astonishing rate – even faster than you lost it. Smart in terms of evolution; not so smart in my situation.

Worse than that were the psychological implications

of starvation mode. Just like with a diet, when foods are banned, your brain obsesses over what you aren't allowed, and for six weeks I hadn't been allowed anything. After my last bout of starvation mode, when I was eleven, it had taken me years to get out of this 'scarcity' mindset. Even within the walls of Rodin House, these rules around food were perpetuated. Fizzy drinks were banned, pizzas were considered treats and if you were fat, or simply a size fourteen like I was, those treats were off-limits to you. Moments like when Miss Naylor batted a cookie out of my hand fed the desire to want to hide food.

All of these desires were undone on arrival at university. My first year at Bristol was the first time I had experienced food freedom. We ate what we wanted and no one judged – or cared – what we consumed. As a result, for the first time in my life, without meaning to, I lost weight existing on a student diet of grilled cheese sandwiches and copious amounts of alcohol. I guess my metabolism had finally normalized after I refused to go on any more diets.

Now, this freedom was gone again. The perpetual thoughts about food and my obsessive scrolling through Instagram food pictures had already warped my mentality back to a place that I thought I'd escaped. Every waking thought revolved around food, and all this restriction had set me up once again for the bodily battles I'd faced back at St Keyes. This time, enhanced by the compliments of weight loss and a physique that I knew I couldn't retain.

*

Once my digestive tract was deemed ready for solid food, I was put on a strict diet of smoothies, soups and other liquids before progressing to bland rice and tofu. At least these were served as real meals, three times a day, and breathlessly I counted down the minutes until the tray arrived in my room. I was desperate to return to my usual fare – dreaming of spaghetti or a perfectly cooked steak. *A piece of chocolate.* But to avoid another bowel blockage, I was fed like a toddler, mashed or milled nursery food delivered in minute mouthfuls. Everything on my plate was chopped and cut up with scissors, reduced to an unsavoury-looking mush and crumbs. I still had a tube in my arm – for various other drips to provide me with further nutrients – and my parents offered to help me, but I was determined to eat by myself.

Desperate for more taste, and something sweet, I begged the nurses to give me an M&M. *Just one, please.* They gave me instead a sip of Gatorade, leaving me unsatisfied and miserable.

Psychologically, I continued to be affected. My obsessional food thoughts only escalated with all the rules and restrictions. Restriction only leads to one thing: unrestricted bingeing, or dreams of it – yet I was still under strict guidelines and asked to mash my food or cut it up with scissors.

These scissors became the legacy of my hospital stay. Within a week of being allowed to eat solid food, I was already on a plane back to England. The doctors advised against it, but I was insistent. It was Emma's birthday in a week, and I wasn't going to miss it. In order to be released, though, from my hospital prison, and allowed to return to England, I had to promise my parents that I would use these scissors carefully and diligently for every university meal. But once I got there, I placed them at the back of my cupboard, never to be seen again. The last thing I wanted to do was pull them out at the dinner table, in front of all my friends, and cut up my food into minuscule pieces like a patient in a geriatric ward. I had longed to return to my previous food freedom. My appetite was unrelenting, and combined with the starvation mode, there was no stopping me.

Looking back now, it was pretty irresponsible to jump back into university life full-throttle. I was easily exhausted and still severely limited in my mobility. On the second night back, when visiting one of my friends, I became so fatigued that I had to be escorted home, despite my insistence that I'd be all right by myself.

Opening the door to my second year house, I was startled that the rooms were all dark. Where was everyone? As soon as I entered the living room, a roar of voices rose up. 'SURPRISE!' Then the lights flashed on.

All my university friends had gathered to welcome me back – and even a friend or two from St Keyes. I burst into tears, stunned and emotional. A surprise party had always been a dream of mine, but this party also meant the final banishment of one of my worst fears: that absence always brought about the disappearance of bonds, memories of good times, and affection. In the past, I had worried that friendships meant more to me than to others. But now,

I saw that love endured. Friendship continued. People remembered me – and cared. There was so much love in the room. That evening, I floated on a wave of ecstasy. All I could see was the beauty in the world.

This heightened sense of appreciation – and acute awareness of the fragility and magic of life – is something that many people experience after coming face-to-face with their mortality, or just facing anything difficult. After coming out of hospital, I had a period of loving life to such an extreme that it felt as if I were a newborn entering the world. I marvelled at the sunlight, the feeling of wind on my skin, the smiles of my friends as they greeted me, and even the smiles of strangers I passed on the street. I stood in wonder and awe of the magnificence of simple things. I was free of the shackles of the hospital bed, free of tubes and drains and needles. I was grateful for everything, from being able to go to the toilet alone to being able to eat.

I had returned to normal but it hardly felt normal to me. Everything I did brought unexpected surprises, intensity and passion. The small excuses I used to make for not doing things – not seeing a friend because I didn't feel like walking twenty minutes – ended. To miss a chance to enjoy the company of a friend was unfathomable. And my level of gratitude for every moment, every experience, was so strong that nothing could get me down. Not even the fact that I hadn't heard from Luke in weeks and he'd been noticeably absent at the surprise party.

*

My first real night out was on Valentine's Day, only four days after my return. I was still quite fragile, but determined not to miss out. A group of my friends were preparing for a celebration together. All eight of us were single, so we decided to pair off for a quadruple 'date' – and end it with a night out at the Lizard Lounge.

My friends and I argued about whether it was wise for me to go, so I agreed to stay off the dance floor and sit near the quiet bar where someone could always keep me company. I couldn't believe how thoughtful they were, not just for insisting on my safety, but because they seemed happy to amend their own partying plans to accommodate my needs.

Getting ready that night was exciting. I was thin enough to borrow clothes from my friends and we spent hours getting ready, outfits thrown on the floor, makeup scattered everywhere. Emma offered to do my hair and I began brushing my fingers through it, just to untangle a few knots, when a big chunk of it fell out. I'd been afraid of this. One of the effects of anaesthesia is hair loss. My fears were compounded by the fact that my scalp was covered with scars and bald patches from my previous surgeries. How much of my hair was I going to lose? And would it grow back?

My friends soothed and reassured me, promising me it wasn't noticeable and that my hair was so thick that it covered everything. On so many of our university nights out there was often some kind of drama – drunken tears, a rush to fetch a box of tissues and fix the eye makeup of the crying girl – and that night, I was the girl whose makeup needed to be fixed. But within ten minutes, my friends had me smiling again, the chunk of hair was in the bin, and I was focusing on the glorious night before us.

The previous Valentine's Day, the girls without dates had all moped together and dwelled on the misery of not being asked out, but this year, I wasn't having it. It seemed absurd that I used to think being single was a valid reason to ruin an entire twenty-four hours. I urged everyone to join me in a reappraisal of Valentine's Day. In its purest form, the day wasn't about romantic love; it was simply about love. And we all have love in our lives, and that deserved to be celebrated. My surprise party, just a few days before, had been a perfect example of this.

To honour Valentine's Day, I banned negativity and complaining. No bitterness or being sad because we were single. My friends acquiesced. My friendship group had always had an uncanny ability to make fun out of nothing – why should this night be any different?

I was determined that everyone should relish the sight of romantic couples on the street – someone handing their date a rose, a girl walking along with an oversized teddy bear, cute couples and public displays of affection. I couldn't believe that year after year, Valentine's Day had brought misery when there was so much to be grateful for.

Since the Lizard Lounge was our last stop of the evening, I assumed there was a chance I'd have my first encounter with Luke since my surgery, and this made me nervous. Would he acknowledge how long I'd been away?

I wondered whether the fact it was Valentine's Day would make seeing him better or worse. And what if he was there with someone else?

A few minutes after arriving, I saw him enter the club – and without thinking, I turned away. When I looked back, he had walked off in the opposite direction. Only an hour later, when we were accidentally positioned next to each other in different conversations, did he say something. 'Hey! Not seen you around in a while. You look amazing – you've lost so much weight.'

I didn't know if that was supposed to be a compliment, but I found it insulting. To focus on my weight loss in the context of what I'd been through seemed demeaning. He must've heard about my surgeries? Did he not care about my health as long as I looked good? To make matters worse, Luke proceeded to recount the names of all the girls he'd asked out for Valentine's Day and been rejected by – apparently forgetting that he'd told me he loved me the last time we'd seen each other, two months before, and that we'd spent the night together.

Wandering off in search of friends, I bumped into Finn, one of the wiser souls from V Block. He was a bit older than the rest of us; he'd been in the Norwegian navy prior to entering the university and had travelled extensively. As freshers, we'd clashed a number of times – he was always complaining about the noise – before he had ultimately admitted that he had a fondness for me. He said I was like an annoying younger sister.

The evening turned starry and shimmering again, now

that I was catching up with Finn and enjoying his company. Behind me, somewhere in the dark, crowded club, stood Luke and his sourness – he hardly mattered any more. Ordinarily, our encounter would have affected me. Or at the very least, would have resulted in a confrontation outside the club – like we had done previously in a drunken spat. But I was impenetrable now; I outright refused to let insignificant events and trivial people have power over my day or even my life. I had context, perspective and gratitude on my side, and some loser wasn't going to take that away from me.

# 30

## Is living in fear living at all?

The months following my hospital stay came with ups and downs, and exhaustion, but my optimism endured. There were academic hurdles, as I tried to make up for lost classes and plummeting grades, but mostly I was under a spell of appreciation for life and a sense of gratitude for my friends, for university life, and for simply being out of the hospital. As the term came to a close, rather than arranging to intern in an office or take summer courses to boost my CV– as many of my classmates were doing – I felt I needed a holiday. Actually, more than that, I felt ready to push myself physically.

Ever since my hospitalization at the age of seven, I hadn't been allowed to do so many things – ride horses, swim, surf, go on theme park rides and rollercoasters. After that first break of my shunt, there was always a feeling that almost anything could break the tube in my neck and land me back in the hospital again. I was afraid of heights, water, almost anything that could potentially put me in danger – or where I might be trapped and not able to quickly see a doctor if something happened. It had been incremental over the years; a slow process that had eroded my confidence in my body and its strength. Bit by bit, I had stopped doing things I loved, and I had lost my voice and spirit.

Now I felt it coming back, as if the hospital experience had reawakened something deep inside me. Landing back in a hospital bed had pissed me off – I had worked so hard to keep myself safe and yet I'd still ended up there. So what was there to lose? I wanted to stop living in fear. I wanted to stop wasting time and start using my body and appreciating it for all it was capable of.

As soon as the doctors allowed me to resume 'vigorous activity', I began going to the gym and I started running. Running gave me mental freedom and an attitude to life that I had never had before – a feeling of steady physical progress. Each day, I did one more minute of running and soon grew stronger. Running gave me such a sense of overcoming all the limitations placed on me during my hospitalization, but more than that, it gave me a place to release a lot of my emotions around it. My university had been less than supportive about my return, asking me to hand in six weeks' worth of deadlines within a week, and running became my way of getting out all the frustration around that. It became my way of dealing with the feelings of injustice and anger I had been experiencing about my lack of health. It became my therapy, and inadvertently it became the solution to the obsessive food thoughts I'd feared. Instead of going back to restricting and dieting, I tried a new approach. I was going to let my body have everything it craved; I was going to throw away my scale and in moments where my clothes stopped fitting, I would remind myself that this was a passing phase and that my body was simply adjusting to eating again. Running helped me remember this. For the first time, there was an emphasis on what my body was capable of, and not what it looked like.

When the summer term ended I returned to Hong Kong for the holidays. With a group of new friends in Hong Kong, I spent the summer pushing myself to the extreme, doing everything that had once scared me. We spent the weeks swimming and paddle-boarding. I even went on a rollercoaster for the first time. We did it all. My friends and I coined it our 'YOLO' (you-only-live-once) summer.

My sister invited me on a hike, and I seized another opportunity to confront an old fear. What scared me about hiking was the feeling of being trapped somewhere or being isolated, with no quick way to escape. This 'fear of being trapped' – which I think was fostered when I was confined to a hospital bed and held there by tubes and drips – had extended to any place that would be hard for me to leave, whether this was an exercise class or social event. On a mountain, there was no way out except to turn back or continue.

By then, I was running twenty minutes continuously – something I had never been able to do before. It was a powerful feeling to gain control of my body and make such strides in my fitness. When my sister suggested a hike in the countryside close to the border of China, ending on a beach with supposedly the 'best pizza on the island', it seemed like an achievable feat. It was one of the more manageable hikes in Hong Kong – a mere three hours – but largely uphill for the first half. The weather that day wasn't working in our favour – blistering heat of forty degrees Celsius and ninety-five per cent humidity – but we weren't deterred.

A ferry and a bus ride later, we found the path. Nestled in the trees, it was a small path that had been flattened by the trekkers before us. The hike began with an uphill climb immediately, as promised, but I assumed there would be breaks and different gradients. Instead, we kept trudging up one mountain slope after another. Eventually we were half-way – ninety minutes in – without hitting a single plateau or downhill gradient. When I looked ahead, all I could see were more mountains and uphill paths.

'When is this going to end?' I asked in disbelief.

'This is the last one, and then it's all downhill,' my sister said, 'and we'll be at the beach where they have the best pizza.'

'You said that before, the last time I asked.'

We rounded a bend and for the first time I could see where we were heading. I was already out of breath from the exertion, and the summer heat, but upon looking down at the sheer drop to the water, my breathing became shallow and quick.

'I need to turn back. I can't—'

'If we turn back, it'll take an hour and a half to get back,' my sister responded calmly, 'so we might as well continue. Either way, it'll take the same amount of time.'

Suddenly I realized that I was trapped – without even the shade of any trees to rest in. My breathing became even quicker and shallower, puffs and pants. In a matter of minutes, I was having a full-blown panic attack. This is what I had feared would happen. My sister desperately tried to calm me down.

I sat down on the path and my sister joined me. I tried to breathe more deliberately, to slow down my breath. Like a mantra, I kept repeating these words in my head: *you knew this was going to be hard, but if you can get through this, you can get through anything.*

I felt stuck, but I had no option but to calm myself down. So I did. Eventually I felt my body relax. My breathing grew slower and steadier. I had faced the thing that I feared – being trapped – and I'd coped. I'd managed. And most of all, it wasn't that bad.

Once we continued our hike, rather than looking down, I focused my gaze on the path ahead and stopped thinking about the time ahead of me, or the path behind me. Staying in the moment, and almost as a perfect metaphor for my journey, I made it to the beach, one small step at a time.

The summer was full of other small moments of triumph. I swam underwater, went to my first exercise class, went wakeboarding and began taking dance classes. My body grew stronger from lifting weights at the gym and from relearning how to box – one of my favourite hobbies as a child. Of course, like back then, it always came with the necessary rules to keep my shunt protected.

You can punch, they can't punch back.

You can kick, they can't kick back.

Regardless, I was taking back control of my body and with each new activity reintroduced back into my life, I felt empowered and more capable than ever before. Each day I was running farther and faster, my fitness improved and my gym sessions began taking priority over my social life. It was almost as if I was in training for something important. Something I knew was coming. A final test of some kind.

# 31

## Is this real?

I awoke to an alarm. A man was standing in the corner of my room. He was tall, broad, dressed in black. He was perfectly still, just as I was. He was standing next to my old wardrobe. He seemed to be looking at me. We were both frozen. I didn't want to move a muscle.

Could he see me looking at him?

Did he know I was awake?

I guessed that it was two or three in the morning – too early for my university room-mates to be awake or hear me. The apartment we shared was in an old building with thin walls and creaking floorboards. I wanted to reach for my phone, to call someone or even just check the time but didn't want to move. I didn't want the stranger to see that I was awake. I just hoped he would leave.

My bed was next to the door, but the man was not too far away. I wondered whether I could escape before he caught me. I shut my eyes. If he saw that I wasn't watching, maybe he would move – or leave.

Blink. Nothing. No sound, no movement. He was still there. My heart was pounding – the loudest sound in the room. Could he hear my heartbeat?

The previous year I'd been told the story of a burglar who broke into the university house next door to ours. The man had entered a girl's room and was taking her belongings when she awoke and saw him. She stayed very still, not wanting to alarm him, but when his back was turned, she grabbed her laptop that was on her bedside table. He whispered, 'I know you're awake,' and promptly exited her room.

This story had haunted me for the entire year, partly because our apartment gave me the creeps. It was safer and more secure than our previous house, but the wind howled through gaps in the windows and there were dark mouldy corners, stained carpets, and creaky floors and doors.

My heart was throbbing through my chest. I opened my eyes again. The man wasn't moving. I was beginning to have doubts. Was he real? In a way, I hoped he was real – that my imagination could play such a trick was even more disturbing. I blinked again, and held my eyes shut for a while, hoping he would be gone when I opened them.

Could this be a dream? Very carefully, so as not to move the duvet, I pinched myself. That's what people did in movies to wake themselves up, so I hoped it would work. But no, I was definitely awake.

He stood still like a statue. He'd paused with his hand

going forward, like a storybook burglar caught mid-act. Still trying to manage my breathing and calm myself down, I noticed the sun had started to slowly peek through my thin curtains. And as the light grew stronger, and glimmered brighter in my room, the man disappeared.

By the time the sun came up, he was gone. I could've sworn he was real – but was I just imagining it?

The third year had begun with more stress than expected. It was our final year. This meant academic pressures, visits to supervisors, an increase in workload, a dissertation to write, and worries about our lives and success after graduation. With persistent questions about what we were doing next, most of us worried about how to find jobs, and wondered what our futures held. The sweet bubble of early university days had burst.

My friendship group had also changed. A few of its members had gone away for a year abroad, and disagreements over housing contracts and other matters had left permanent rifts. Our old habits of partying and drinking excessively were replaced with nights in the library and job applications. Many of the girls had serious boyfriends now, and spent the rest of their spare time paired off with them. We gathered to see each other only for the occasional birthday party and coffee.

I had also begun seeing a boy, but it was a long-distance relationship. Rory was pensive and opinionated, curious about the world – and intellectual. Our differences had attracted me to him. He was studying for a graduate degree in London and had a full-time job in Bath, which meant we only saw each other once a month or so. I had met him on Tinder. Passionate about politics and the law – two subjects I knew very little about – his fervent rants about policy were a refreshing change from the idle banter that my friends existed on.

Another difference between us: while I had grown into an unrelenting optimist, Rory had a pessimistic and un-trusting view of the world, often stating his belief that you should 'fuck people over before they fuck you over'. For some strange reason, this didn't concern me. Given my unwavering romantic nature, I felt lucky to be trusted and allowed into Rory's life. His unique ability to moan about the smallest of things also fascinated me. We were opposites, and I supposed that meant our attraction was real – after all, opposites attract, right?

Most of my time was spent studying and writing. I had tried not to pay attention to the fact that much of the psy-chology course had been extremely monotonous – training us for clinical trials, statistics, drugs and research. The degree was more technical than human-based. While my passion for psychology had slowly drained, I remained persistent that all this would change when I began studying for my master's, when the subject would grow more practical.

Then, just four months before graduation, I had a mod-ule that was the most intriguing by far. We began learning from practising psychologists who introduced us to all the different forms of therapy and branches within the profession. Each week, a different psychologist would talk about their work with actual patients – real people with real conditions and disorders. In the past, I had often wandered into lectures late or missed them entirely without giving it much thought; now I went to every lecture, and never arrived late. When discussions ran over, I stayed until the end, not wanting to miss a thing.

One week, the lecture concerned the impact of physical illness on an individual's psychology. The lecturer, an older woman with a serious demeanour, described how psychologists in this sector were brought into hospital wards to work with the chronically or terminally ill; individuals who had severe diseases or life-threatening conditions. She explained how they counselled the patients about how to adjust to their new life with a health condition, or even prepared them for death.

Sitting near the front, I became aware of emotions welling up inside me. Just hearing descriptions of the hospital environment and about the lives of chronically ill people took me back to that environment in my mind, as if it were a separate place or alternate universe where I had once lived but had forgotten existed – or tried to forget. I stopped taking notes. Suddenly I was eleven again, that small girl in the big white hospital bed, surrounded by specialists and surgeons and nurses, and I understood why I had behaved as I did – how angry I was, and sad, and scared. I had never let any of these emotions fully surface, but stuck in that front row of the lecture theatre, it felt like for the first time, I didn't have a choice.

As the lecturer kept talking, it was like watching a slide-show of my own memories and experiences, each flashing before me, each causing a different sensation. Sure, the doctors had treated my physical conditions – and performed surgery after surgery on my body to make corrections that had kept me alive and allowed me to live a full life. For years I had struggled to find ways to deal with my physical scars, to hide them, show them, talk about them, and even how to warn boys about them. I thought they were my biggest problem. But there were other scars to consider – the ones inside me.

I felt restless in my seat. My legs began bouncing nervously and my heart raced. My feelings were beginning to overwhelm me. The lecturer continued talking.

'As a working psychologist, you will face the daily stigma that psychology is only for crazy people,' she said. 'This is very common in a hospital setting, because nobody really wants to be there – or wants to face what they are experiencing. The standard response, when I tell them I'm a psychologist, is "I'm not crazy", or they suddenly begin screaming, "Why me, why me?"'

These words rang inside my head, louder and louder. I couldn't hear anything else. *Why me... why me... why me?*

I had trouble catching my breath. Trapped in the middle of a row, my tears were impossible to hide. The lecturer noticed me, and caught my eye, and I tried to hide my embarrassment. With Freddie next to me, I muffled my sobs and sat through the rest of the lecture with my head spinning out of control. I tried to refocus on what the woman was saying but it was impossible. A Rolodex of images was spinning in my brain – things I hadn't thought about in years. Lying on the carpet with Mrs Wright standing over me; being wheeled into the emergency room in Los Angeles and all the people bleeding and crying around me; the loneliness of the ICU; the moment visiting hours ended and I began crying hysterically as my parents got up to leave; the quiet and emptiness of the hospital nights; trying to reach for the call button; waiting for the dogs to visit; the moment my heart stopped and I left my body, when I died, and the sound of my mum's shrieks and cries in the room. All those moments, locked away inside me, were rising up, demanding to be remembered.

As the lecture came to an end, it was agony waiting for the students in my row to stand up and leave. I hoped that Freddie wouldn't try to talk to me – or ask me any questions. I avoided eye contact, and when our row was clear, I picked up speed and ran out of the theatre. I found a bathroom and locked myself in a stall, trying to breathe and calm myself down. Freddie would still be in the building, wondering where I'd darted off to, but I thought if I stayed in the stall long enough, he would give up looking for me.

I wasn't even sure why I was crying – why now, why so suddenly? Taking slow breaths, I began to steady myself and gain more control over my emotions. 'I'm going to be all right,' I reassured myself. 'I'm just going home to bake.'

Baking was one of my favourite pastimes. It was something I had always loved to do at school, passing the weekends at St Keyes in cookery classes and then later, at university, making brownies, cookies and cakes for my housemates. I knew this would distract me. As soon as I got home, I dug out all the ingredients and a recipe. I knew it would make me feel much better. My mind was focused on that task. *Chop the chocolate into small bite-size pieces.*

I pulled out a rolling pin and started pounding on a chocolate bar, slamming it into little bits. Thumping the bar down on the tabletop, my mind went back to the lecture, the way the psychologist had talked about people with chronic illness and again, I started to think about the hospital – the days and weeks and months of fear and loneliness, living with tubes and wounds. No privacy, no control. If I had asked, could anyone have been able to give me an answer – *why me?* But there was no answer, no explanation. Suddenly, all the unexpressed anger of those years filled my head, whirling and swirling, each new churning thought moving too quickly to be processed, each one sending me into a wilder sense of panic.

I grabbed the rolling pin and began smashing it against the table, over and over. With each smash, I wanted to break the panic, break the spell of anger, and return to my old self, my old normal Michelle, how I used to be – just an hour before.

'What's all that noise?' It was Tess, my closest friend in the house. She'd walked into the kitchen and was looking at the rolling pin in my shaking hand. 'What's wrong?' she asked. 'Are you OK?' Unable to speak, I went back to banging the pin on the table, hoping she wouldn't notice that I was crying.

'Michelle, stop!' She grabbed my arm, mid-air, and began hugging me from behind. After I'd collapsed into her, sobbing, I felt a new surge of emotions: sadness; anger; confusion. Only a murmur came out of me, drowned out by my tears and panic. How could I begin to explain? It seemed that I was crying about being in the hospital – but which stay, which surgery, what year?

I went back to my room, trying to put the episode out of my mind. I chose to chalk it up to a bad day, to hormones, something I'd eaten, or lack of sleep. I felt certain it would be gone when I awoke the following morning. But the next day, as soon as I was fully awake, a stream of memories and thoughts rushed into my mind. I was overcome with a sadness I couldn't escape, just like the day before.

For the next few weeks, these thoughts were with me wherever I went, whatever I did. The only way of coping was shutting down. I went to lectures and trudged home, went straight to my room and cried. Some days, I would miss my lectures because my eyes were too swollen and red from crying all morning, so I would stay in my room and cry all day in bed.

I would eat chocolate, burn candles and watch old episodes of the TV show *Full House*. Someone had recently given me a box set of the series as a joke, and that became my escape – just as it had been in hospital.

Rory was an escape, too. I spent many hours texting him. His complaints about his excessive course-load or annoying colleagues felt simple and solvable, unlike my monstrosity of problems that I couldn't begin to understand or address. I still believed that I only deserved 'convenient love' – love that would vanish if things became difficult or complicated. My disappointing experience with Luke had only confirmed this, so I'd decided not to mention the hospital at all to Rory.

When my housemates asked how I was or why I was sad – wondering what had happened to the loud, laughing and smiling Michelle they were used to – I couldn't really explain because I didn't understand it myself. I knew it was about the hospital. I knew it had something to do with my operations, but I didn't know how to process my emotions or make any sense of them. I just wanted the whole thing to be over and decided just to wait it out. But after three weeks, I was still sad and still crying, often muffling the sound of my sobbing with my pillow, and spending more and more days in my room. The only time I left my room was for more chocolate – and to check the front door of our apartment to make sure it was closed and locked.

My old habit had returned. I knew it wasn't rational, but much like scratching an itch, it was an urge I couldn't control. My housemates noticed this new tic, and found it peculiar that I needed to double-lock the front door when I was home alone during the day, and they would complain about how annoying it was. I tried to hide it from them, debating how I could double-lock the door for long enough to feel secure, yet unlock it before my house-mates started returning from class.

That's when the nightmares began. I would wake in the middle of the night, or early morning, having dreamed that

I was in surgery and paralysed by the anaesthesia and was unable to move. Repeatedly, I re-lived the moment that I'd died in my hospital bed and, waking in a panic, I would sometimes see the man in the corner of my room, the stranger.

*He isn't real. He isn't real.* It was a hallucination.

Turn the lights on. See for yourself.

Then I heard his voice. He was calling my name. It was getting louder and louder. I was afraid to leave my room.

'Michelle, Michelle... Michelle.'

'No! No! No!' I cried out. I thought by repeating the word over and over, and speaking out loud, that I could ground myself in reality, and make the illusory disappear. Finally, in a moment of courage and curiosity, I propped open my bedroom door in order to see the front door.

Freddie was standing there.

'What the fuck are you doing?' I cried out, trying to hide my weird behaviour. 'You freaked me out!'

'I just came to see you.'

'Why are you just standing outside someone's door? That's really creepy...'

'I knocked,' he said calmly. 'You probably just didn't hear me.'

He looked alarmed. Since the episode in our lecture, I hadn't seen him in more than three weeks. When he'd called to make plans, I'd told him I was ill – or busy. We would normally see each other every day. My tear-stained face and red eyes were a giveaway that I'd been crying, and now it was too late to pretend otherwise.

And it was time to tell him the truth. About everything – the lecture, my nonstop crying, the memories of surgeries and hospital stays.

'Why didn't you tell me?' he asked afterwards.

'Who wants to be friends with someone who cries all day?' I said. 'You told me once that I laughed more in a day than you did in a month. Where did that person go?'

He sat in the corner of my kitchen and held my hand. His face showed a mixture of confusion and disappointment that I hadn't felt comfortable enough to talk to him about it. 'Oh Michelle…' he moved closer and folded me into his arms. He rubbed my back and held me tight. 'I'm not your friend because you laugh and smile all the time,' he said.

'As much as I love that about you, if you want to spend the next six months crying, I'll still be here for you – and so will all the friends that matter to you. You will get back to your normal self, I'm sure of that. But first you need to ask for help.'

I knew he was right.

# 32

## Am I still me?

Within hours of Freddie's visit that day, I looked up the name of a psychotherapist, Dr Stone, who was trained in psychodynamic psychotherapy – a form of treatment that I had studied in class. It's a more long-term approach than cognitive behavioural therapy (CBT) and relies on a study of underlying causes more than just fixing symptoms.

As soon as I booked my first session, though, doubts began to creep in. Mostly I worried about whether I truly needed help or deserved it. People lose their limbs, go through wars, have cancer, suffer from poverty, disease and untold other miseries in life – as evidenced on television every day. Here I was, complaining about something that happened ten years ago. It seemed almost embarrassing. As I waited for my therapy appointment, I felt myself becoming more and more nervous. And I'm sure this had something to do with the stigma around therapy itself.

In England and Hong Kong, particularly, therapy carries a heavy stigma and facing that felt like an identity crisis. Going to see a therapist meant admitting I wasn't 'normal', a label I had yearned for throughout my life. I didn't need another reason to feel defective. Another thing: Dr Stone's office was located in a nice area of town, much too nice for the bulk of students to live in, but close enough so that it was possible that I could run into random friends or acquaintances on my way there. That worried me too. Even though I was about to graduate with a degree in psychology, and hoped to pursue graduate work that would lead to a qualification as a psychologist – that was my vague plan, anyway – the idea that I would be caught on my way to a therapy appointment scared me. I thought of St Keyes, the cruel jokes about Harriet and the derogatory comments about any girl who had 'issues'.

The prevailing attitude was summed up by something my dad once said. When I was still in high school, I asked him if he knew any psychologists whom I could intern or do work experience with over the summer, and he immediately replied, 'No! Why would I know any psychologists? I'm not crazy.'

Entering the book-lined office, I was greeted by Dr Stone, an older woman with long brown hair that framed her face. She had a kind face but it was devoid of feeling or warmth. Later, I would come to think of this as 'the psychotherapist's expression' or rather, no expression. She had been trained not to react to any information that a client might reveal. It was meant to encourage patients to open up more freely in an accepting clinical environment, without criticism or judgement. But instead, I found staring at a blank face a little unnerving.

We began the session and I told 'my story'; mostly the litany of operations and hospital stays, the uncertainty that I felt in regard to my health, which had led to a lack of confidence in my body. Was my body really on my side and making my life better – or was it always tripping me up with complications and problems and terrible surprises? It was still too soon to discuss my hallucinations and flashbacks. I knew the point was to tell her what was concerning me, but those things I couldn't discuss. Surely vocalizing them would make them more real? So I just began with why I had come that day, and relaxed in the knowledge that I was in safe, experienced hands. Perhaps, most of all, I was being productive and proactive in seeing her, and attempting to make positive changes.

Very unexpectedly, though, Dr Stone had a diagnosis before the hour was up. She was very confident and very certain. There was no doubt: I had *post-traumatic stress disorder* (PTSD), she said.

'What?' I said, taken by surprise. 'I can't have PTSD. I didn't have a trauma. What happened to me wasn't even a big deal. It's not like I had cancer.'

'You said that before,' Dr Stone replied. 'You said what happened to you wasn't a big deal, that you didn't have cancer. But you had a brain tumour, didn't you? Why is there such a distinction in your mind between a tumour and cancer?'

'My tumour wasn't cancerous. Cancer is serious and long term,' I said. 'My brain tumour was benign, removed and is gone!'

I left her office with more questions than I'd had when I arrived. Having studied psychology, I knew the basic symptoms of PTSD, but as soon as I got home I looked them up again. My symptoms did match up: the sense of suffocation or feeling trapped, the re-experiencing of the traumatic events in the form of flashbacks, which could be hallucinations or repetitive distressing images and sensations. But it felt like an exaggeration – I truly did feel like a hypochondriac now. What I had been through shouldn't result in such an intense reaction, surely?

It seemed far too serious, and far too debilitating. I thought of PTSD as something that happened to war veterans and victims of sexual abuse. In hospital, I was told that I was a survivor, not a victim. In school, everything was treated like it wasn't a big deal, so that was what I believed. At university, I was seen as a positive, strong person, the light of the party. Or at least, I had worked hard to be. Essentially, Dr Stone was saying that I'd made light of deep wounds from trauma and blithely skipped over the process of true recovery. I just wasn't sure that could be true. Unless everything I had been told was a lie?

Over the next three one-hour sessions, while I cried my eyes out, Dr Stone tried to convince me that I had been lying to myself. She said that I had dismissed my true feelings in the environment of the hospital because they didn't seem appropriate – and they weren't helping me to survive. My body was healing and that took priority. People in a crisis or going through trauma, essentially in survival mode, tend to shut down emotionally just to make it through.

She argued that survival mode continued when I left the hospital, at St Keyes, where it wasn't safe to have feelings or show them. The school culture itself was brutal and bullying – not a smart place to show vulnerability. And there might have been a fear of reprisal at the school for the way Mrs Wright had treated me, keeping the administration from appearing to be concerned about my health when I returned. In any case, the message was loud and clear: everybody was to act like nothing had happened – including me.

My survival at St Keyes required that I gloss over my deepest feelings, my outrage and sadness. The *why me?* Now it was time, she said, to start being honest about how I felt.

This made sense, and I nodded my head a lot while Dr Stone explained her view, but being honest about how I felt was a lot harder than I had even imagined. I'd been rewarded time and again for being upbeat; now, to call my experience a 'trauma' required a reconsideration of almost everything I felt about myself. It flew in the face of what I had always believed: that gratitude was the path to happiness, not wallowing in misery and bad memories.

At the same time, whenever I thought about the hospital, I began to cry. I sat with tears streaming down my face in Dr Stone's office – and cried all the way home. She continued to reassure me that often these feelings got worse before they got better – but how much worse, and for how long? My mind fought this new approach, and kept fighting it. The emotions that I was beginning to feel were strong and confusing. I wasn't sure that I could ever make sense of them, process them or make them disappear.

In subsequent sessions, Dr Stone helped me to untangle how I was feeling. While I cried and talked, for the first time I felt like I could vent without burdening my friends. For the first time, I felt like I wasn't being judged. I found comfort in knowing that she must see more extreme cases throughout her day. Surely she was accustomed to hearing much worse. Slowly, I began to see that most of my responses and attitudes about my operations weren't really my own, or genuine. They were sentences that had been said to me with the best of intentions, and which I repeated. *I was lucky. I should be grateful I survived.* My real feelings were buried beneath a wealth of learned phrases. *You should be so proud of yourself for overcoming adversity.*

*Michelle, you're such a strong girl!*

Placed in a confusing situation at a young age, I naturally believed what the people around me were saying. Besides, I liked being a strong girl – and didn't want to be seen as a victim or unlucky. When people gather around the hospital bed of an eleven-year-old girl, they will do anything to make her feel better, to keep her feeling positive, even in the grimmest situation. And while this may be beneficial in the moment, it results in keeping the child from adequately processing the series of events for herself, or even coming to experience her truest, deepest feelings. With each comment, I felt more pressure to uphold the image of a 'survivor'.

With each psychotherapy session, I trawled through my emotions with a fine-tooth comb, looking for the real feeling underneath the stories of courage and resilience that I had been telling myself and everybody else for years. And what I found wasn't so admirable or courageous.

Deep down, I was furious. Deep down, I didn't feel so lucky. The overshadowing memories of my childhood were things that had happened in hospitals – and left me with big scars all over my stomach, neck and head. I had never spent a carefree day. I had never played happily on my bike. I was always worried about damaging my tube, falling and hitting my head, or worse. Each day had brought stress and a feeling of responsibility for my health, and trying to decide what to tell my parents. I'd hidden my migraines and lied about my feelings, not wanting to reveal my pain.

As I sat there, ranting to Dr Stone, the anger eventually turned to sadness. It dawned on me that my childhood had never really existed. This became painfully obvious when one of my university friends, Spencer, a jovial person, had an upcoming neurology exam and asked if he could practise on my housemates. When he showed up at our apartment to do this, Tess immediately looked at the stethoscope around his neck.

'What's that?' she asked, pointing to the instrument.

I was stunned. There were actually people in the world who didn't know what a stethoscope was? 'Are you kidding?' I asked her.

'No,' she replied. 'What is that thing?'

My amazement deepened. 'But you must have seen one before,' I persisted.

'Maybe,' she said. 'I think so. I just didn't know what it was called.'

'You really have never heard the word "stethoscope" before? You didn't wonder what it was called, when you went to the doctor?'

'But I can't remember the last time I went to the doctor,' Tess replied. 'Maybe a couple of years ago.'

Now, I was baffled. 'Wait—' I said. 'So you've not had a cold in a year?'

Tess looked confused. 'You go to the doctor for a cold?'

People really do grow up in different homes, different worlds. There wasn't a detail of a doctor's office or hospital environment that I didn't know the word for – whether it was cerebrospinal fluid, spina bifida or peritonitis. I had no clue what it was like to not question my health or go to a doctor for every little query or grumble, 'just in case'. This conversation reminded me how truly alone I was in my experiences. And how each visit to a medical office triggered more worry in the people around me. That was the other thing that made me sad: how much hurt and fear my health had caused in my family. To this day, my parents are hyper-aware of my health and safety.

At the suggestion of Dr Stone, I began to keep a journal.

The following passage was written after my fourth session and demonstrates the raw feeling and scattered state of mind of someone struggling with PTSD:

A large thing for me today was realizing that I feel like my childhood was taken away from me, my innocence – and the fact that I had to deal with mortality at a young age. I guess I didn't think it affected me because I'm not scared of death. But in a way, it's not very normal to not be scared of death. And if I'm not scared of death, then why do I have paranoia and fear? Is it purely about experiencing pain? I don't know, I sort of came out of therapy with a heavy weight that I couldn't shirk, I just felt generally down. Only when I was kept busy with other people's problems did I not think of my own. The difficulty is that with my lack of lectures, it's getting harder and harder to avoid my thoughts.

I'm also having a great sense of being misunderstood and feeling like there's no way I can explain it even if I wanted to. That no one understands me because they don't understand my past, so they can't understand what I'm going through at the moment. I tried to explain it to Freddie today and before I could even begin, I didn't know whether I should. I didn't think he would understand. I feel like eventually everyone is going to tire of having me around, of having to put up with me and my low moods. I mean, it's not fair to them. I've been isolating myself from people and not explaining why. Such a large part of what everyone says they like about me is that I'm always so happy and positive and smiley – without that, I'm just not sure…

Tess said today, 'I know I'm not going to understand what you're going through, and I'm going to give you your space to think everything through, but if you ever need to talk I'm always here.' I mean, how perfect can my friends get? I'm angry, though, about the fact that I couldn't experience any of the things my friends did growing up. I'm angry that I look back at my childhood and all I can remember is homework and hospital. I can't remember running around, having fun and just being carefree.

This anger made me very apathetic today, just about everything and life. I didn't care about work. I didn't care about my dissertation. I even stated I didn't care if I dropped out right now. I'm starting to not care about a lot of things.

\*

Until therapy started, I had still been seeing Rory – and texting him a lot. We'd been seeing each other for two months before the subject of my operations, scars, or any else health-related had come up. We were planning a visit – and I knew he would be staying over in my room. In a fumbling way, I'd explained that I'd had surgeries and then waited for him to follow up with questions, but he asked nothing. And later, when he saw my scars for the first time, he said nothing. So I tried a different approach. When we were talking, I began a story with, 'When I was in hospital...' thinking that might prompt him to ask me something. The first time I tried this, he didn't seem particularly curious. I began to wonder if he felt awkward or was just too self-centred to care.

One morning, when we were lying in bed, my head resting on his chest, Rory raised the subject himself. 'I've been meaning to ask you, what were your surgeries for?'

He nodded along as I started to describe the beginnings of my medical drama. I couldn't see his reaction, which helped me to keep talking. He said nothing, and didn't even move. His hand was lying still on my shoulder as I continued to elaborate. When I got to the part about my intestines being 'punctured', Rory became agitated.

'*Ewwww!*' he said suddenly – the universal sound of disgust. 'OK, you can stop – I'm squeamish!' Maybe he meant the procedure disgusted him, and not me personally, or even my scars, but it was hard not to feel hurt. He was only hearing a medical description. I had lived it. But, as usual, I tried to focus on the positive. Maybe he didn't feel my medical history was important to our relationship. Maybe he wanted to be with me regardless – and he saw the stories of operations as ancient history. But I knew I was kidding myself.

# 33

## What's my identity?

Denial. Some say it's inevitable; some even say it's wise. After all, humans would never consciously put themselves in the path of pain – would they? That's what you do in therapy. Day after day, week after week, pain and more pain. I would wake at midday and my crying would begin almost as soon as my eyes opened, sometimes before. I would surface from my room only to use the toilet, then would return to bed and cry again. Around 3 pm, I would look for some chocolate in the cupboard and return to bed, still crying. By 6 pm, my eyes would be sore and swollen – looking as if I'd had an allergic reaction. I would leave my room for a wet facecloth to place over my eyes to relieve the throbbing pain.

I had never been a 'crier' before, not really – not compared to other girls. At St Keyes, my friends had challenged me to watch both *The Notebook* and *Titanic* without a single tear – which I could accomplish easily. But now I found myself contemplating whether there was a maximum capacity that a person could cry, and what my own capacity was. Each day I would cry for six hours, almost straight, terrified that the sadness had no end and the rest of my life would be spent this way – if my eyes didn't give out first. They seemed permanently swollen and under pressure, almost as if every blood vessel in them might pop.

Initially I found it cathartic to cry my eyes out, but before long, it became excruciating. And just getting myself to Dr Stone's office became a struggle. As I walked to my appointment, I would prepare myself to remember and discuss the worst moments of my life in infinite detail. And after I left, the sad effects would sometimes linger for six days. Just as I was beginning to feel normal again, and crying less, it was time for the next session. I would battle myself for the few hours beforehand, hoping to come up with a good excuse not to go. On the walk there, I wanted to turn back halfway through. I was just starting to feel better – why would I want to feel worse again?

My ultimate low came just a few days before the Easter holidays. My housemate Tess, who had been doing all my grocery shopping for me, had gone out and wasn't expected back until the evening. But I had run out of my previously endless supply of chocolate. I crawled out of bed and decided to walk to the supermarket that was located on the triangle, next to the infamous Lizard Lounge. I never gave my appearance a thought. I was just desperate for chocolate.

My hair was pulled back in a four-day-old bun, a halo of messy stray hair floated around my head. My eyes were so sore that they couldn't tolerate my usual contact lenses, so I found a pair of old glasses. Making this combination worse was my outfit: trackies with a gaping hole in the crotch and a short black T-shirt that barely covered my boobs. I was someone who had never left the house without a bra, but for the first time I was too tired and sad to bother.

I ventured out for provisions – three bags of chocolate – and was returning with a shopping bag in hand when suddenly, finally, the reality of my situation hit me. *Who and what had I become?* It wasn't my appearance that was the problem, but my complete apathy towards everything. This was simply mirrored by my appearance.

The old me, the real me, the Michelle that I had been my entire life, was never an apathetic person. She had personality, drive, ambition – or simply, purpose. And now, I was unrecognizable – not just visually, but emotionally. I was an empty shell, and for the first time I could feel it. I had hit rock-bottom. I was drowning in self-pity, and it clouded who I was. As soon as I had this realization, as if by magic, I started to feel better. I couldn't do this any more. I needed to stop wallowing. I needed to help myself.

Upon my return home to my family in Hong Kong for the Easter holidays, I felt happier and more stable. Away from my university room, which had turned into a pit of tears and despair, my mood definitely changed. I was no longer engulfed in sadness. The only time I felt bad was when I thought about therapy – and imagined returning to Dr Stone and continuing to tell and re-live my saga. One night, I admitted to my parents that I'd been feeling lost. I had kept them in the dark, but now I needed their help. I was feeling lost and confused, and began wailing.

'You're allowed to be angry,' my dad said. 'All these years, I couldn't understand how unaffected you were. These feelings are inevitable.'

This small and simple phrase gave me the permission I needed – not to be a saint or survivor. I went on, explaining how I also felt sad that I'd missed out on a childhood, and how alone I felt! That no one could fully understand.

As I continued to talk, my hysterical wailing quietened and I became calmer.

'Sometimes you have to ignore things to be able to live your life,' Dad said.

'But what about this pattern of denial that I supposedly have?'

'It's not denial,' he said. 'You were happy before, you can be happy again. Sometimes over-analysing things can leave you with lots of explanations but no relief.'

Graduation loomed, and my future. Therapy had led me to understanding my problem, but hadn't offered ideas or answers to help me change things – and feel better. I had one final therapy appointment, and I sat there with one very simple question:

'What next? Where do I go from here?'

Dr Stone's answer: 'This is your life now. We just learn how to manage it.'

No, I couldn't accept that. I *wouldn't* accept that.

# 34

## What happens now?

My relationship with Rory had crumbled again. He'd said he was tired of all the 'drama' – which made me laugh, given how much drama I'd been keeping from him. We had gotten back together shortly after I ended therapy. He never knew why I had changed my mind about our first break-up as I hadn't told him about therapy or my PTSD; in fact I had barely ever spoken to him about myself or my life. At times he'd accused me of being naive or gullible, of wanting to see the good in everything. 'One day,' he said, 'someone is going to hurt you so badly that you will become sceptical like the rest of us.'

Perhaps it had been wrong to keep so much from him. I had never given the relationship a true chance. Once it ended for the second time, we were both insistent it was better that way. He said it was important to him that we stayed in touch, and we did – eventually becoming closer as 'exes' than we were as a couple, texting every day. I had been planning my twenty-first birthday party for months, long before any of the PTSD symptoms had started, and I was determined not to let anything get in the way of that night. It was scheduled for just two days before graduation, at a restaurant in London. I had invited my extended family, some old friends from Hong Kong and St Keyes, many more from university – and even Rory. I had planned every detail of the event. And I was spurred on by the prospect of having everyone I loved in one place, one room – something that rarely happened, if ever. On the evening of the party, as I looked around the crowded private dining room, I couldn't help but glance at Rory every so often, to see whether he was having a good time – or fitting in. It was just two weeks after we'd broken up and we hadn't seen each other, despite the constant messaging.

After champagne and toasts, and after dinner was served, Rory had to leave early. He found me before he went. 'I have to admit that I'm kind of jealous,' he said. 'I've never seen people care so much about one person. There was so much love in the room.'

It wasn't like Rory to be so complimentary – or open. I stood silently, not really knowing what to say. 'The sad fact is,' he went on, 'I can't say I have one friend who has the level of friendship with me that you have with each of the people in this room. Any one of my friends would throw me under a bus in a hurry. I've come to accept you will always be a happier person than I am.'

It was a striking statement to make about himself – and his life. I cared so deeply about my friends, and looked after my relationships, because I knew what it was like to lose them. And it was true, even in the darkest times, when my whole life seemed like an utter mess, that I saw the best in others – or tried to. I guess this made me seem 'happy' to Rory.

As I watched him go, and returned to the rest of the revellers, I thought about his remarks. This party wasn't just another birthday celebration; it was my first. I had always had a superstition around celebrating my birthday – that actually enjoying it would jinx my luck.

Turning twenty-one was an anniversary: it was ten years since my heart line had flattened on the hospital monitor. I may have come back to life that day, but some things hadn't made it with me. My childhood innocence; that naïve dismissal of mortality. People often ask young kids, 'What do you want to be when you grow up?' and children reply with enthusiasm and certainty about how they're going to achieve their dreams. They don't see the obstacles and challenges, or even the technicalities involved. What I learned ten years ago was that not everything *just works out*. Wishing doesn't make things so. And not all dreams come true. It was a hard lesson, and in many ways I was still experiencing how hard it was.

Two days later, I officially graduated. I guess in part, I was proud that I'd completed my dissertation despite my wavering mental health. That somehow I had accomplished something despite the odds being against me. But I was ready to say goodbye. Returning for the ceremony seemed unnecessary – a formality. I was ready to leave behind the place where all my problems had surfaced. But seeing me graduate was important to my parents, especially my mum.

She beamed with pride as I walked carefully to the stage and accepted my certificate and then posed for the official graduation photo. It was as stereotypical as you could imagine – cap, gown, happy parents in the background. It ended up being a fun day; a final goodbye to a place where I had learned a lot and come into my own.

# 35

## Is this what happy feels like?

The first year out of university wasn't easy – for me, or for many of my friends. There's such a hype around graduation – that it's meant to be the happiest day of your life. But instead mine brought a load of uncertainty. I suppose the world expects you to be certain about your goals, and to pursue them at full-throttle. But instead, I felt even more lost than I had before. I was now living in London, a dream I had had ever since moving to England for boarding school, and while I was glad it was happening, it didn't bring the certainty that I expected.

For years I had kept anxiety about my future at bay with my narrow focus on becoming a psychologist. This focus had been my coping mechanism. My life had a greater purpose – and sense of direction – thanks to that ambition. I sometimes wonder if this ambition was a result of the St Keyes mentality: I had been raised in a school environment of restless, driven overachievers. But now I wasn't so sure. To be a psychologist, I would have to be sorted myself – and I was far from having my life sorted. My scars and emotional conundrums would have to be explored and made peace with. But I had tried conventional therapy and found it limited. In fact, I considered the experience a failure. Instead of empowering me to work through my problems, Dr Stone had wanted me to just accept them and settle for mediocre standards in terms of what my life should be. It seemed counterintuitive – and not the type of therapist I would want to be.

There were certainly other, easier paths in life. Some of my friends were hoping to become accountants or lawyers, or to work in the City. They were applying to graduate schools and knew the proper paths. I didn't know where to begin, where to apply or what to do. But when I ran through a mental list of other professions, none of them seemed half as rewarding as psychology. At my core, I still found humans and human behaviour more fascinating than anything else.

Imagine being able to help people with their lives, and make them feel comforted, understood and happier? I had trouble comparing that to working in a bank or in marketing or advertising – the routes psychology students often seem to take. I just wished I could be a different kind of psychologist. One who didn't make it so clinical with the strict fifty-minute guidelines, the stone-cold expressionless face and repetitive reactions. Did a job like that even *exist*, and if so, what was it called?

Everywhere I went, at each social engagement, people asked me pointedly about my future plans. What was next? And instead of saying that I was planning to be a psychologist, I found myself lying, pretending to be so busy that I was unable to think or answer. Before long I settled on an answer that seemed to shut down all inquiries: 'I'm taking a gap year and going travelling.'

Yes, it was a way of shutting down the questions – but perhaps it wasn't such an awful idea? Maybe it's what I needed, to take the pressure off – or at the very least, to delay any decisions I needed to make. It was decided: I would go travelling in January. But in the meantime, I had three months to kill.

Keen to avoid excess time for my thoughts to run wild, I started booking on a variety of psychology-related courses – anything I could find. New models, new approaches... new me?

I booked onto a total of five courses. I'd started with an interest in hypnotherapy, but with each discovery came several more new terms I hadn't heard before: Time Line Therapy™, neuro-linguistic programming, coaching... the list went on. The majority of these courses were free 'taster days', so there was nothing to lose. But this time, I was going to do things differently. I refused to accept the possibility of a client discovering ten years later that this stuff didn't work, so I needed to try it myself first. If it was better than therapy, then the results must be better too – and I was going to test it, personally. After all, I still had an excess of issues that needed fixing.

I began researching various treatment centres and practitioners, looking for someone who was trained in working with people with trauma. I was still extremely sensitive and continued to cry often. I found a clinic that used a number of different treatments that I'd never heard about – all of them hypnotherapy-based. The office was located on Harley Street, the most prestigious street for medical procedures, which gave it more credibility in my mind – although I have to confess I was still very sceptical. Over the phone, when I asked how many sessions I would require, I was alarmed that the therapist said I would only need one or two.

How could that be true? I'd tried psychotherapy for over four months and had come away feeling worse. This particular technique – 'Havening' – could cure my symptoms in two hours? I was beyond curious.

After making an appointment, I was asked to fill out a pre-session questionnaire. It was ten pages long and asked many broad questions and took me six hours to complete. This already seemed a more effective approach than traditional psychotherapy, during which the basic questioning and description of my emotional problems had consumed the initial four sessions.

On the phone, the hypnotherapist explained that trauma occurs when you have an inability to escape your environment and the nervous system doesn't know the difference between what is imagined and what is real.

He used the example of imagining biting into a lemon. Even the mention of it provokes the physiological reaction of your mouth salivating without the stimulus – the lemon – being present. He explained that that's what had happened with my traumatic memories. A distraught reaction occurs when these memories, real or imagined, are re-lived physiologically.

From the perspective of hypnotherapy, the conventional 'talking therapy' that I had undergone had only embedded this further. Recounting and re-living these memories had caused the re-running of neural networks, which activated the PTSD symptoms. And each time I recounted and re-lived the experiences, it made the wiring of these circuits stronger. He had a remarkable ability to answer every question that I had with scientific data. I was still sceptical, but for the first time in a while I was hopeful.

The office on Harley Street looked like any other doctor's office – cold, professional, minimalistic. I began to feel nervous, preparing myself for the inquisition that usually occurred in a therapeutic setting. Instead, the hypnotherapist, a middle-aged man, started the session by asking about my specific symptoms, and then he asked what my worst memory was.

'The day I died,' I said.

As I began to describe it, tears filled my eyes. He stopped me from going further.

'You don't need to explain what happened,' he said.

'Unlike other types of therapy, this isn't going to be painful. I'm not going to make you re-live it – you've done that enough. How about we make you feel something different instead?'

I was confused. How was this guy planning to help me, if he didn't know what happened?

He explained that saying those four words – 'The day I died' – had already triggered the mental pathway, and provoked the pictures and images that I associate with this event to run through my mind. As he put it, the event itself wasn't the problem – only my perception of it, and the negative meanings and emotions that I had attached to it. His plan was to interrupt the pattern. He would introduce new associations, soothing gestures, soothing sounds. I would be asked to think of 'the day I died', hug myself and sing 'Happy Birthday'. Then I would be asked to move my eyes from right to left and back. These lateral movements would induce delta waves, provoking good feelings while I was remembering the worst day of my life.

He told me to think about the event – and asked me if I was picturing the event happening. I said that I was. He then asked details about these pictures. He didn't want to know the content, just the physical details – how big, how bright, 3D or flat, black and white or colour? This was all to do with the way in which my brain stored these memories. Each of these details related to how my brain encoded the feelings connected to them. Then he told me to imagine flinging these mental images to the corner of the room. Did that feel better or worse?

Definitely better.

Then he asked me to imagine pushing them to the other side of the world, and then falling off a cliff into the depths of the ocean. So I imagined myself as a small girl again in a hospital bed. Then I pictured tossing that image out to sea.

But then I grew agitated. 'Stop!' I called out, with my eyes closed. 'I can't get rid of the memories. I won't. I need them!'

'What do you need them for?' he asked.

'If I got rid of all this pain, and these memories, it would be disrespectful and ungrateful to the children who died. Or the other children who were in the hospital with me – the ones who never got better. It's not right to try to forget what happened. I need to feel grateful to be alive.'

'You will always have your memories and you will always have your gratitude,' he said. 'What you'll be doing is getting rid of the emotions associated with these memories – not getting rid of the memories themselves.'

He explained that this new technique, 'Havening', alongside neuro-linguistic programming (NLP), would alleviate my symptoms. These were called 'psycho-sensory' approaches. I would later learn that these processes, sometimes referred to as 'submodalities', are believed to work because our memories are stored and recalled via mental images that we have daily, but that we are not often conscious of. It can be best demonstrated by asking a participant to imagine a house, then to put it to the side for a second and imagine a car. What will physically happen in the participant's mind's eye is they will have literally moved the house to the side, either left or right, because the unconscious mind takes us literally. This can also be done with memories.

It was important, the hypnotherapist told me, that I let these old memories and feelings go. I hadn't been able to move on because I'd wanted to remember the children that hadn't gotten a chance to grow up. Unconsciously, he said, I was living my life with these experiences in the forefront of my mind – demonstrated by the fact that these images were physically at the front of my mind when I recalled them. He explained that by doing that, I had held onto my own pain. Living free of these associations, he said, was a way to honour and appreciate life in a genuine way, rather than continuing to inflict pain on myself.

I was worried about something else, and raised it with him. 'If this process works,' I asked, 'how can I be a psychologist?'

'Well,' he answered, 'what's the purpose of being a psychologist?'

'To help others.'

'And is there another way you can help others?'

I thought for a second. 'Yes. Yes, there is.'

A great weight was suddenly lifted off my chest – and replaced by a sense of freedom. *I didn't have to be a psychologist*. Other burdens were gone too – things that had been keeping me in a painful place. At the end of a two-hour session, the hypnotherapist asked if I had any further questions. I thought for a second, and said, 'This is what happy feels like. I had forgotten.' In a matter of minutes, my whole life seemed to have been returned to me.

Walking down the road after leaving the therapy office, I felt joyous – light, buoyant, relieved, exhilarated. It seemed almost too good to be true. Was I really fixed – without even that much of a conversation? What amazed me most was that throughout the session, the therapist had no clue what had happened to me or what memories I was letting go of. These didn't need to be described or explained. To say the experience baffled me would be an understatement. I felt a sudden urge to call all my friends, or even my parents, to tell them about this incredible session, but I didn't want to raise their hopes – or my own. What if all these good feelings vanished a day or a week later? *But I need to tell somebody.* So, on my way home I called my sister.

'So the weirdest thing just happened to me...' I began. I really didn't know how to describe the last hour – I was very aware that describing the actual process would make me sound slightly ridiculous. But I tried, and she listened very carefully. At first she seemed just as sceptical as I had been.

We were still talking when I arrived at my apartment in London. Inside the door, I found an envelope with my name on it. It was a huge envelope, and heavy, almost bursting at the seams. When I opened it, I found my entire medical record from America, a bulky 500-page document. I had contacted the UCLA medical centre several weeks before and asked for my complete records for my doctors in London. And here it was.

The timing seemed almost spooky. The pages held the account of all my various traumas, written in medical jargon and other code. 'I can't believe it,' I said to my sister. 'Of all days – when I finally feel better.'

'Don't you dare look at it!' she cried out. 'If this session worked, you're just going to undo everything! Don't even open the package. You're going to find out things you don't need to know. Just hand it straight to the doctors.'

But as soon as I hung up the phone, I opened the package and before I knew it I was sitting on my bed, reading. Flicking through the records, it astonished me how much detail there was. I turned back to the beginning, slowly reading each line.

Alone in the apartment, I nestled under my duvet and read. I had initially decided I would only look at a few pages, but it was like a bedtime story that I didn't want to finish. I kept going, rationalizing that this was the proof I needed about NLP. If I could get through the reading of my medical file without losing it, I would feel more confident that the Havening session had worked. Hours passed, and I made my way through the entire document, reading the intricate details of each operation, the daily accounts of my hospital stay – and the doctors' comments.

I read about the day they discovered the brain tumour, the day that I flat-lined. I read about my tricks, my bad attitude and my 'depression'. I read it all without one moment of sadness. Not a single tear.

It wasn't until I woke up the following morning, still

feeling happy and unburdened, that I was convinced something profound had occurred.


Confidence is a process. You don't just wake up one day
feeling fantastic about yourself. It's a journey that involves
baby steps, ups and downs. It's rarely a straightforward
story. But I tried to build on what had already begun. In the
months that followed that first session, I trained to become
a 'change work practitioner', which is what the therapists
who practise NLP, Havening and Time Line Therapy™
are called. The initial session had brought a lot of my
physical symptoms to an end – the crying, the flashbacks,
the hallucinations – which in turn made my problems seem
more manageable. My healing had begun.

Part of what my dream had always been was to give
back. I believed it was an essential part of being grateful
to everyone who had helped me when I was little. I began
volunteering at Great Ormond Street Hospital in London.
It was the perfect way of getting closure on a lot of my own
experiences. Initially, I worked in the corridor, guiding lost
parents to where they needed to be, and then eventually I
moved onto the ward. The children would tell me about
what they were missing at school or how they felt left out
and wished they could see their friends. The nurses often
seemed exhausted and underappreciated.

It was on one of my volunteer shifts at the hospital
that I saw a therapy dog arrive at the ward I worked on.
I stopped to talk to the dog's owner, an older woman with

rounded glasses and a gentle smile. I wanted to convey to her how much the dogs had meant to me all those years ago, in my own hospital experience. I told her a little about the dogs that had visited me, what they looked like, and their names. It made me smile just to think of them again.

Just as I was about to leave, she reached out to say something. 'Thank you for stopping me today, and for thanking me,' she said. 'You never know whether you're actually making a difference – or what kind of impact a visit is having. But more importantly, thank you for having a conversation with me. People rarely notice me when I'm with my dog. They're looking down the entire time, and only see my ankles.'

My job at Great Ormond Street gave me great solace. And it gave me a chance to say a lot of things that I needed to say – not just thanking the doctors, nurses and volunteers, but giving advice to the children, and trying to comfort them with words I wish I had been told. It was my way of rewriting history, by helping others and making their experience different to mine.

A lot of paths in my life began to converge, or come full circle. Even Rory returned. He had seen on Facebook that I'd started a life coaching business, and upon seeing my first YouTube video, he contacted me. In the video, 'How to Talk to Boys About Your Scars', I mentioned different ways that I'd done this, and although he wasn't mentioned specifically, Rory recognized himself in one story. While recording and releasing the video, it had never occurred to me that he would watch it – much less message me about it.

'I remember when I got that text,' his message read, pinging up on my screen.

Slightly embarrassed, I wrote back to him instantly and apologized – saying that I could have handled things better when I told him about my scars. But he said they had never changed his perception of me, or made me less attractive to him. The entire time we were dating, Rory had never used the word 'attractive' to describe me, and because of my insecurities, I believed he had never thought it.

His reassurance felt nice, but mainly because I knew I no longer needed it. My scars had begun to mean more to me than any man's seal of approval in terms of beauty. In facing my past, they had become symbolic of my story – a representation of a struggle I had faced.

Having completed my training, I was getting started with my own clients and had cancelled the majority of my travelling plans. Instead I decided to squeeze my gap-year plans into a month. I went to Australia with Nadia, one of my friends from university. It was an eye-opening and liberating month. In many ways, I had carved this time out to be the childhood I never had – or at least the teenage years I desperately wanted rather than the academic rigour I'd had.

Nadia was very sociable and outgoing. I was bold and daring in a way I had never been before. We spent days at the beach, swimming in rivers and pools, kayaking, surfing, hiking to little ponds and waterfalls. We made friends wherever we went. Since my 'YOLO' summer, I had continued to face my fears, but now being in Australia took it to another level with spiders, sharks and jellyfish everywhere and more dangerous and poisonous than in any other place in the world. By this point, my coaching training was ingrained in me. Everything was simply a mindset and I was equipped with the tools to handle any fear, wobble or insecurity I faced.

For the majority of time we were in our swimsuits, which is what sparked a question from Nadia. It caught me off-guard. It also changed the path of my career.

'Why don't you wear bikinis?'

# 36

## Am I ugly?

It was a sunny day in Florida as I stared out across the pool. I was sitting in a bikini and six months had passed since Nadia had put that question to me. I had flown to Florida for a coaching retreat – the first time I had gone anywhere alone since my interviews at Oxford. I was a coach now.

Coaching had been the perfect fit for me and provided the solution to everything that hadn't sat right with therapy. Coaching is more future-focused than therapy. Therapy asks what's wrong and how you feel about it, whereas coaching asks what you want to be different and how you can make that happen. They were different methods; different processes designed for different people. Therapy might help one, but coaching will be the solution for another. It was nice not only to know there was an alternative, but also to provide one.

My friends were kind and supportive, but didn't fully understand where this 'new me' was coming from. That was partly why I'd decided to go on a coaching retreat – to meet people who were interested in coaching but not coaches themselves. And sure enough, within the first few hours, I had bonded with a woman called Hayley. She was much older than me, with a completely different life – kids and a husband. She was loving and tough, supportive and ambitious, and it was because of her prodding that I had put on a bikini and was wearing it by the pool.

Goal-setting is part of coaching. Goals take time – and you have to plan for them. You decide on what you want, make it as specific as possible, assign a date to it, and then you take action towards your goal while believing with a hundred per cent certainty that it's going to happen. Goals like 'I want to be happy' are not goals. These are states of mind, feelings that you can gain in a second. A goal requires planning and patience.

The goal I had set for Florida was to wear a bikini for the first time since I was ten years old. I was pretty determined, but the night before I left for the retreat, I realized that a crucial step in the 'taking action' part of goal-setting had been forgotten: I hadn't bought a bikini. So I did some panic-shopping online, and a next-day delivery later, a box of bikinis arrived at my flat. When none of them fit, I decided to shelve the entire idea.

'It's OK,' I told myself, 'I've completed a lot of goals. I can let this small one go.'

In Florida, I told Hayley about my foiled plans – how

nothing had fit and that it was a silly idea anyway. The next day, she whisked me down to the hotel shop and stood outside my changing room until I found a bikini that looked good. I put a sundress over it and we all went down to the pool.

I had so many awful memories that went with swimsuits – and it's probably the same for most women. As I walked to the pool, I imagined the judgemental stares of the other hotel guests, and the looks of shock and pity. I put on a cold exterior – another skill learned at St Keyes – so I wouldn't show that I was vulnerable, but inside, I felt ten years old again. To keep myself from backing down, I whipped off my dress as soon as I arrived at the pool. Then I walked around the corner – to join a gaggle of women.

Hayley was beaming with pride and clapping, and embraced me with hugs. The other women seemed confused, so it was explained that this was the first time I'd worn a bikini as an adult. 'Oh,' the women said, looking straight at my face and not at my scars, and I was applauded again, and congratulated – and then, in just a few minutes, the hubbub was over and the conversation moved back to a discussion of lunch, and where we were going, and what we wanted to eat. Nothing had changed. In fact, everything was exactly the same. I didn't want to stand out or be different or pitied. I just wanted to be like everybody else.

'Hey, what does your tattoo mean?' Hayley asked, looking at my wrist and seeing a little blue bow that I'd had inked there.

I explained that I'd been to Japan during the summer holidays of my first year of university and visited hot springs, where it was customary to be naked. There, a little girl had stared at me all day, making me more and more confused, and frankly insecure.

Later I'd asked my friend, 'Was it because I'm fat?' and it was only at that point, seven hours afterwards, that I realized what the little girl had been staring at: my scars. My natural assumption was that it was my fat – something every woman worried about – and I had completely forgotten about my scars. It felt liberating – and normal. Something I had tried to attain my whole life.

I had gone from never talking about my scars or surgeries in my last year at St Keyes, to talking about them so much in the first year of university that I got a tattoo of the number thirteen. And this felt like balance. Forgetting my scars for those seven hours reminded me of something I'd forgotten: I'm more than my scars. I'm more than my body. To commemorate that moment, I got a tattoo – a blue bow made out of circles, because I had come full circle. The placement on my wrist signified that everything I touch is affected by these experiences; but the bow is on the side, because my scars are not the centre of my world but a side-story.

'Wait,' Hayley said, 'there's something I don't understand.'

'What?'

'You were wandering around the hot springs naked?'

'Right,' I said.

'Then why was a bikini such a big deal?'

It's funny how it sometimes takes an outside perspective to see through your own insecurities. Hayley was right. My problem wasn't really with my body. My problem was the bikini – two flimsy pieces of fabric. For so long I'd believed that my life would begin when I lost enough weight and loved my scars enough to wear a bikini. I believed that if I could accomplish that, I could achieve anything.

And I was right. But only because I believed that a bikini stood in the way of everything. Now, in a bikini, without the weight loss and with my scars on show, I felt exactly the same as I'd imagined I would all those years ago when I used bikini photos as my motivation for weight loss.

But this pride, this euphoria, it wasn't from weight loss – it was from finally being myself, authentically, exactly how I was and how I looked right now, not in five, ten, twenty, thirty pounds from now. Ignoring all the societal standards for what a bikini body looked like – I was doing it. Fat. And it was more empowering than I could have ever imagined. I was deviating from the norm – the norm I had so desperately wanted to live by. But being realistic, I *wasn't* normal. Not my story, not my scars, not me – so why was I trying to be?

My body had never been the problem. After all, how many people with my medical record have the privilege of even *having* a body? I was alive and I wasn't going to spend a moment more of my life letting what I looked like stand in the way of my dreams.

*

'Hi, I'm Michelle Elman and I'm a body confidence coach,' I said to two tall, beautiful women.

Coaches are urged to find a niche and I had been toying with the idea of one. The problem was, I had never heard of this as a field, and according to Google, there were no 'body confidence coaches' – only a few emotional eating coaches, but to me, that wasn't the same. I wanted to create a niche where eating and exercise didn't come into coaching but instead physical insecurities were simply seen as manifestations of internal insecurities – much like how the issue of my scars had resolved itself once I confronted my past. I would be establishing a new niche in coaching, and I was worried this was being a bit too gutsy. Everywhere I looked there were women with body confidence issues, but if I chose this as my field, would I have any potential clients?

I decided to go to a networking event, where I would meet people from various industries and professions, in order to give my idea a try.

'Body confidence? That's so cool!' said one of the women at the event. 'What are most people insecure about?'

'It's usually their legs,' I said, 'especially before a night out.' I hadn't done any kind of research; I was merely speaking from my experience of being surrounded for years by women discussing a litany of insecurities.

'That's exactly what I was thinking!' she replied. 'Just yesterday I was trying to convince her,' she nudged her friend, 'to wear a skirt even though she said she thought her legs looked ugly. What else? Tell us more.'

I felt an adrenaline rush. I didn't need a doctorate degree or experience doing clinical trials. I had given advice sessions about body confidence issues my whole life. Now I simply had the techniques to create a change in mindset that anyone might need.

'The main insecurities are brought out in the bedroom,' I continued. 'Especially with your stomach hanging out, if you're on top.'

'Oh my god!! Yes! That bothers me so much!' the woman agreed – and then another person tapped me on my back.

'Hi! I just heard what you were talking about and I'd love to know what you think about…'

Then another, and another.

In the space of ten minutes, I had drawn a crowd. Each person had more questions than the last, and eventually all of them asked for my business card. Before I knew it, I had a niche, clients and something important to help them with. I'd been hesitating over a photo of myself in a bikini, taken in Florida a month before. I had yet to post it on any social media, but knew I wanted to do something with it. Volunteering at Great Ormond Street had made me realize how many children grow up with scars; I can't have been alone in my body woes? I can't have been the only one who worried about scars? As the author Brené Brown says: 'Shame only exists in silence.' I couldn't have been the only one who lived with shame around their scars. I had just discovered the hashtag #bodypositivity on Instagram and there were so many women embracing their bodies, but not a single one that looked like me. There wasn't a single account talking about scars, and I was determined to be that voice. In a place where all bodies were being embraced, why wasn't there one with scars? I didn't want this body positive space to exist without scarred bodies being represented. I'd spent my whole life asking, 'Why me?'; now I was asking, 'Why not me?'

Several weeks later, having posted the photograph of myself in a bikini on Instagram – to launch my body confidence campaign, using the hashtag #ScarredNotScared – I returned to my phone an hour later to see the post had gotten over 400 likes, the most I'd ever had, and a number of bloggers and YouTubers that I'd followed for years had seen and liked it. As the days passed, I continued to watch the numbers grow, then I hit publish on a blog article I had written for the *Metro* a website where I had already been blogging. The next day the *Daily Mail* got in touch with me to do a story, but warned about the nature of their comments section.

'Are you sure you want to go ahead with this piece?' the editor asked. 'If you do, I would urge you not to read the comments section.'

I had already prepared myself for the worst, and spent an hour thinking of all the terrible things anyone could say about me online. And I could only come up with one thing: that I was fat and shouldn't be wearing a bikini. The word 'fat' was not going to stop the momentum of my campaign. Fat wasn't an insult to me – it was simply a fact, a descriptor. I knew I was fat, and anything else they might say to me, I was sure I'd said worse to myself. I'd received a comment on my initial blog post the previous day, while I was with my friend Emma about to go swimming: *Nothing wrong with wearing a bikini just because you have scars... however not when you are morbidly obese.*

My fifteen-year-old self would have gotten a bag of chocolate after reading that remark, and spent the next few months actively trying to pretend I didn't care. But then I imagined another fifteen-year-old girl reading my article. I envisaged her reading it, maybe considering wearing a bikini for the first time, and then reading the comments and realizing I was only one voice in a sea of people who thought bodies like mine shouldn't be allowed to wear a bikini due to my size. I had to do something. I needed to address my weight.

As Emma and I were about to go swimming, it seemed like the perfect time. Standing on the side of the pool, I decided to film another video in response to that comment. I read the comment out loud, then kissed my hand, slapped my arse and jumped into the pool. When I posted it on Instagram, just like the previous post, an overwhelming number of likes poured in. I checked back a few days later and that first comment had been deleted. Unheard of in the world of trolls.

Then the first negative comment on the *Metro* came in:

*Don't think they are staring at your scars love, I think*

*they've always wondered what the Michelin man's wife looks like.*

I decided to respond:

*I'd be honoured to be the Michelin Man's wife... He seems like a nice guy. Also, 'Michelin Man and Michelle Elman' has a ring to it. Thanks for taking the time to read my article Tim ♥*

Within a few minutes, I received a notification that Tim had replied:

*Glad my daft comment washed over you like water off a duck's back! Just had a look at your Facebook page and you're clearly well above comments like mine, which is the way it should be. You know what's what. Impressed by your response to me too! :)*

The following day, Buzzfeed, The Huffington Post, *The Independent*, and Bustle all got in touch. By then it had spiralled – there were articles about me in *Cosmopolitan*, *Seventeen*, Women's Day, *The Mirror*. I knew it had gone worldwide when my cousin in Israel tagged me in a post from Portugal, where the hashtag #scarrednotscared had been translated to #vaitercicatriz. I was contacted from America by *People* and *The Today Show*.

Meanwhile, messages were pouring into my social media accounts and people were baring their souls, telling their stories – many for the first time. I was suddenly in a position to speak out about my own experiences and become a role model of sorts – a position which seemed odd considering it wasn't that long ago that I was wracked with insecurities myself.

I thought back to that Havening session, before which I'd believed being a psychologist was the only way to help people, and now here I was, changing people's minds with a simple photograph. I suddenly realized the importance of embracing your story. It had been liberating for me, and somehow it seemed to be liberating others. But it wasn't me, it wasn't my body: it was the realization that you aren't alone.

I thought back to my childhood and how happy I would've been to see someone with scars in the magazines, and that's when I realized the impact of a photo – and more importantly representation. If I could've seen some-one like me, maybe – just maybe – I would've felt included or even accepted. Maybe I wouldn't have had to battle my body so much. Maybe I would've realized being normal isn't everything. Maybe I would've realized that I didn't just deserve 'convenient love', but real, true love.

Somehow, with one photograph, I had stumbled across my passion and my purpose – I wanted to create a space for these people to be heard. But how? First, I had to be honest with myself and give myself the help I had never felt I deserved. I didn't just deserve it – I had earned it. I felt my whole life's purpose was to help others. I was doing that. Now it was my turn.

I'd found a new therapist, one trained in a more holistic approach, combining my new coaching beliefs with spiritual work that included meditation. A lot of our sessions revolved around healing my inner child and learning to comfort myself as an adult, and through one of these meditations, I felt the urge to have a conversation with myself that was long overdue.

I sat down, pen in hand, and began writing.

Dear eleven-year-old me,

I am so sorry for all you've been through, and more than that, I'm sorry that you ever questioned that you did something to deserve this. You didn't deserve any of this. There is nothing that you did to make this your fault. There is nothing you could've done to prevent this. I know you were told that everything happened for a reason, but that's not true. Sometimes awful things in life happen to good people. Please know you are a good person.

You are going through a really scary point in your life right now and I know you might not feel ready to talk about it, but please talk to someone. You aren't alone. There are so many people in your life who love you and want to help you, but they can't unless you ask for help. I know that can be scary and you want to be brave and strong and make everyone proud, but you're only eleven years old and you can't know all the answers. I know you want to bury all that has happened in the past and pretend like it never happened, but it did happen. And it sucked – it's OK to admit that. Vulnerability is bravery, and asking for help doesn't make you any less resilient.

You have just gone through something that very few people your age will understand, and that might make your friends awkward around you or uncomfortable in talking about what you've been through, but know that this isn't a reflection of you. Finding friends is a difficult process, and one that can take years. Your popularity is not a sign of your worth. You are worthy and lovable, and as you grow up you will find some amazing friends who will have your back through each and every hospital visit. When you get ill, they won't disappear but will instead hold you closer and make sure you know that you are loved.

I wish I could hug you and tell you that you will never go back into hospital again, but that isn't true. You will go back into hospital again, but please go live your life as if you won't. Living in fear is worse than not living at all, and I want you to make the most of the body you were given while you have the chance. I know you are already hating your body and the scars that lie across it, but please believe me when I tell you that those scars are what make you beautiful. Understand that even if you hate your body, your body loves you. Your body fought for you to keep you alive and breathing every single day, so please stop fighting your body. You are on the same team.

Your scars might make you different, but being different isn't a bad thing. Being 'normal' and wanting to fit in are overrated, and your unique story is what is going to make you shine. You will learn to love your story over time, but for now, do your best to be nice to yourself. You deserve that.

I love you so much
**Michelle.**

# EPILOGUE

'How do I become more confident?'

This is the question I have been asked daily, if not hourly, on my Instagram over the last four years. It's a simple question, with a not-so-simple answer. It's a question I've come to dread, because no matter how I answer it, I will always be oversimplifying. A lengthy response reflects the length of time it took me to achieve this so-called 'confidence'. A brief response would imply that it was easy to get to this place – and now that you've read my story, you know this couldn't be further from the truth.

That's why I wrote this book, because no 300-word Instagram caption, or 1,000-word blog post, could adequately portray how complex and messy the journey to self-acceptance is. There are twists and turns, and most importantly, times when everything goes downhill. Confidence is not an uphill journey and not all progress looks like progress at the time. Oftentimes, progress actually looks like failure in the moment. The pivotal moments in my story – the small decisions I've made to become more confident – only become important with hindsight. The honest answer to that question is that there is no way I could be the person I am today without every single event that took place in this book.

When responding to the question, I often emphasize the small steps. It's a clichéd answer when given in an Instagram message, but now that you've read the book, you can see for yourself. It was a moment in a hospital bed, when I refused to take my life for granted. It was a decision to be more inclusive in a fashion show. It was the realization that my body still worked. It was deciding to take myself to therapy. It was deciding to tell my friend that I had a dream of wearing a bikini. Those small steps are what are important and what make you more confident. Those small steps show that confidence is achievable for anyone. My baby steps will not be the same as yours and my journey will never be the same as yours, which is why I'm wary about handing out generic 'confidence advice' – but what I do know is that I didn't become confident until I realized that confidence was an option for me.

All through my teenage years, my goal was simply to be less insecure, to hate myself just a little less, because I believed every human lived with insecurities and that it wasn't an option to actually love yourself. How wrong I was! Loving yourself is an option; loving your body is an option and you have to choose that option for yourself. Your journey of self-acceptance is exactly that: yours.

Want to wear a bikini? Great, go buy one first. Much like me, most people forget that vital step because they forget about the baby steps.

Want to wear those short shorts? Great, wear them around the house first. You need to remember who you're wearing them for – yourself. Your happiness is more important than other people's opinions.

Want to get comfortable in the bedroom? Great, start brushing your teeth naked first. You can't love your body if you don't know what it looks like. Get comfortable with yourself naked, and then worry about someone else seeing you.

Want to be as confident as your body positive role model? Great, read their captions, see their happiness and absorb all their 'BoPo' goodness, but don't compare yourself to them. You're seeing the end of their journey, whereas you're only at the beginning of yours. You're at the fun part!

The person who becomes the most confident is the one who is consistent in their pursuit of it. The person who achieves self-love is the one who is kind to themselves when they feel they least deserve it. The person who accomplishes self-acceptance is the one who loves themselves in the moments when hating themselves is the easiest option.

This book is my way of saying: it's your turn.

# ACKNOWLEDGEMENTS

During the times when I lost faith in this book, I would imagine writing this section of it – so to finally be doing it is incredible. I can't believe that all of this came from a twelve-year-old girl writing an autobiography as an assignment for English class; but to get it from there to here was no easy feat and couldn't have been done without the help of so many people.

Martha Sherrill, thank you for undoing years of being told that I was a bad writer and for helping me find my inner storyteller. Anna Hogarty, thank you for holding my hand through this entire process and always matching my passion. This ride wouldn't be as fun without you. To everyone at Madeleine Milburn Literary Agency, thank you for making me feel so supported and for doing all your magic behind the scenes – I can't thank you enough. Thank you to Ellen Parnavelas and everyone at Head of Zeus who has worked so hard to make my dream a reality. From the first meeting, you all made this such a special process!

Michelle Zelli, my mini-miracle, there is no way I would be the woman I am today without you. Thanks for being such an example and loving my inner child, even when I couldn't. Sophie Pugh, thank you for always being there, being my 'surrogate boyfriend' and always laughing when I yell 'turnip'. Thanks also for putting up with all the nights you used to come home to me sobbing while I was writing this book. Uncle Michel and Auntie Angele, my second pair of parents, you both hold such a special place in my heart and always will.

Thank you to the body positive community – there are so many of you now, each one a massive piece of my journey in embracing who I am. Special thanks goes to Megan Crabbe and Hannah Witton, who gave me space in their books before I got the chance to have one of my own! Thanks for helping me keep the dream alive! And thank you to every child I met in hospital along the way – I might not remember your names but I will never forget your faces.

Thank you to Dr Lazareff and Dr Peacock; I literally wouldn't be here without you, and this book certainly wouldn't exist without you. I wish every doctor had as much care for their patients as you two do. To Christie and Amy, thank you for making my life in hospital bearable. Thanks for being the reason I have some good memories from that time.

Thank you to my sister for being the first person to teach me to stand up for myself and raise my voice. Thank you to my brother for making me stronger and loving me, even when you hated me. To my mum, my fierceness is all down to you. Thank you for always doing your best, looking after everyone and saving my life. And thank you to my dad who believed I was a writer long before I did, and told that twelve-year-old to publish her school project. It might have taken twelve years, but look Dad – I did it!

# FURTHER RESOURCES

**My Social Media Accounts**

| | |
|---|---|
| Instagram: | @ScarredNotScared |
| | @BodyPositiveMemes |
| Twitter: | @ScarredNtScared |
| YouTube: | Michelle Elman |
| Facebook: | Michelle Elman |

**Body Positive Instagram Accounts**

This is by no means an exhaustive list but one that is intended to get you started. Each of these people is someone that I follow personally and in some way or another has helped me along my journey.

Aarti Dubey – @curvesbecomeher
Alex La Rosa – @missalexlarosa

Alysse Dalessandro – @readytostare

Allison Kimmey – @allisonkimmey

Amy Wooldridge – @amyeloisew

Ana Rojas – @powertoprevail

Anna OBrien – @glitterandlazers

Bertha Chan – @curvasian

Brittany Burgunder – @brittanyburgunder

Callie Thorpe – @calliethorpe

Charli Howard – @charlihoward

Cheyenne – @goofy_ginger

Chloe Elliott – @chloeincurve_

Clare Sheehan – @becomingbodypositive

Colleen Reichmann – @drcolleenreichmann

Dana Suchow – @dothehotpants

Danielle Galvin – @chooselifewarrior

Danielle Vanier – @daniellevanier

Danni Gordon – @chachipowerproject

Denise Bidot – @denisebidot

Ella Endi – @nakedwithanxiety

Eff Your Beauty Standards – @effyourbeautystandards

Essie Dennis – @khal_essie

Felicity Hayward – @felicityhayward

Gabi Gregg – @gabifresh

Gia Narvaez – @thesassytruth_

Grace Victory – @gracefvictory

Harnaam Kaur – @harnaamkaur

Honorine Elizabeth – @honorcurves

Imogen Fox – @the_feeding_of_the_fox

Janny Gate – @jannylivesunapologetically

Jessie Lupinetti – @jessie_lupinetti

Joeley Bishop – @thevagaggle

Kelly Knox – @itskellyknox

Kenzie Brenna – @omgkenzieee

Kitty Underhill – @kittyunderhillx

Lottie L'Amour – @lottielamour

Megan Crabbe – @bodyposipanda

Meghan Kacmarcik – @sundaesforthesoul

Meghan Tonjes – @meghantonjes

Morena Diaz – @m0reniita

Nicolette Mason – @nicolettemason

Olivia Campbell – @curvycampbell

Paola Zuccaro – @chubbybabe_

Rebekah Taussig – @sitting_pretty

Ruby Allegra – @rvbyallegra

Sarah Vance – @sarevance

ShiShi Rose – @shishi.rose

Simone Mariposa – @simonemariposa

Summer Innanen – @summerinnanen

The Unedit – @theunedit

Victoria Welsby – @bampowlife

Virgie Tovar – @virgietovar

Whitney Way Thore – @whitneywaythore

## Body Positive Books

*Body Positive Power* – Megan Jayne Crabbe

*Big Girl: How I Gave Up Dieting and Got a Life* – Kelsey Miller

*Health at Every Size* – Linda Bacon

*Hunger* – Roxanne Gay

*Shrill* – Lindy West

*The Beauty Myth* – Naomi Wolf

*The Dance of Anger* – Harriet Lerner

*The Gifts of Imperfection* – Brené Brown

*Things No One Will Tell Fat Girls* – Jes Baker

Or come join the Body Positive Book Club on Facebook!
(www.facebook.com/groups/BodyPositiveBookClub)

To

_Yvonne_

From

_Two - Two_

BroadStreet Publishing
Racine, WI 53403
Broadstreetpublishing.com

# BIBLE PROMISES *for You*

ISBN 978-1-4245-5029-6

Compiled by Michelle Winger | literallyprecise.com
Designed by Chris Garborg | garborgdesign.com

Printed in China

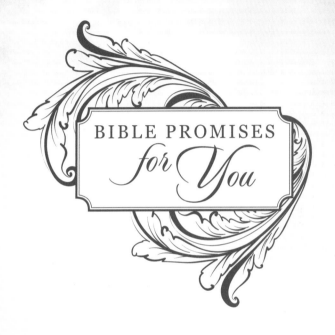

BIBLE PROMISES
for You

**BroadStreet**
P U B L I S H I N G

$\mathscr{E}$verything you need to get through each day can be found in the promises of God's Word. *Bible Promises for You* is a topically organized collection of Scripture that is designed to help you recognize who you are, and who you can be, when you embrace the truth of His Word. Each theme declares a promise you can claim over your life and Bible verses to help you grab hold of that promise.

Find the inspiration and encouragement you need in God's Word. His promises are for you every day!

# CONTENTS

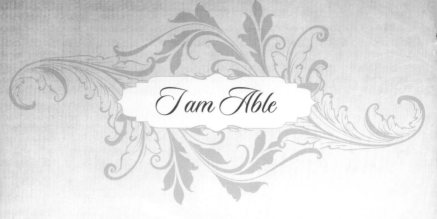

# I am Able

We are not saying that we can do this work ourselves.
It is God who makes us able to do all that we do.

2 CORINTHIANS 3:5 NCV

Take a new grip with your tired hands and strengthen
your weak knees. Mark out a straight path for your feet
so that those who are weak and lame will not fall
but become strong.

HEBREWS 12:12-13 NLT

"My grace is sufficient for you, for my power is made
perfect in weakness." Therefore I will boast all the
more gladly of my weaknesses, so that the power of
Christ may rest upon me.

2 CORINTHIANS 12:9 ESV

We can rejoice, too, when we run into problems and trials, for we know that they help us develop endurance. And endurance develops strength of character, and character strengthens our confident hope of salvation. And this hope will not lead to disappointment. For we know how dearly God loves us, because he has given us the Holy Spirit to fill our hearts with his love.

ROMANS 5:3–5 NLT

After you have suffered for a little while, the God of all grace, who called you to His eternal glory in Christ, will Himself perfect, confirm, strengthen and establish you.

1 PETER 5:10 NASB

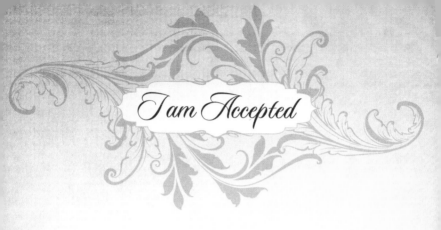

# I am Accepted

The Father gives me the people who are mine. Every one of them will come to me, and I will always accept them.

JOHN 6:37 NCV

Before he made the world, God chose us to be his very own through what Christ would do for us; he decided then to make us holy in his eyes, without a single fault— we who stand before him covered with his love.

EPHESIANS 1:4 TLB

If God is for us, who can be against us?

ROMANS 8:31 ESV

Here I am! I stand at the door and knock. If anyone hears my voice and opens the door, I will come in and eat with that person, and they with me.

REVELATION 3:20 NIV


I've redeemed you.

I've called your name. You're mine.

When you're in over your head, I'll be there with you.

When you're in rough waters, you will not go down.

When you're between a rock and a hard place,

it won't be a dead end—

Because I am GOD, your personal God,

The Holy of Israel, your Savior.

I paid a huge price for you...!

*That's* how much you mean to me!

*That's* how much I love you!

ISAIAH 43:1–4 MSG

# I am Adopted

You did not receive a spirit of slavery to fall back into fear,
but you have received a spirit of adoption. When we cry,
"Abba! Father!" it is that very Spirit bearing witness with
our spirit that we are children of God.

Romans 8:15–16 nrsv

The Lord will not abandon His people on account of His
great name, because the Lord has been pleased to make
you a people for Himself.

1 Samuel 12:22 nasb

I will not abandon you as orphans—I will come to you.

John 14:18 nlt

A father of the fatherless and a judge for the widows,

Is God in His holy habitation.

God makes a home for the lonely;

He leads out the prisoners into prosperity.

PSALM 68:5-6 NASB


But when the right time came, God sent his Son, born of a woman, subject to the law. God sent him to buy freedom for us who were slaves to the law, so that he could adopt us as his very own children.

GALATIANS 4:4-5 NLT


I will bring the blind by a way they did not know;

I will lead them in paths they have not known.

I will make darkness light before them,

And crooked places straight.

These things will I do for them,

And not forsake them.

ISAIAH 42:16 NKJV

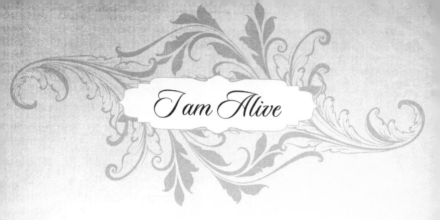

# I am Alive

Dear friend, listen well to my words;

tune your ears to my voice.

Keep my message in plain view at all times.

Concentrate! Learn it by heart!

Those who discover these words live,

really live; body and soul....

Keep vigilant watch over your heart;

that's where life starts.

PROVERBS 4:20–23 MSG

I am the resurrection and the life. He who believes in Me,

though he may die, he shall live.

JOHN 11:25 NKJV

Sin...doesn't, have a chance in competition with the aggressive forgiveness we call *grace*. When it's sin versus grace, grace wins hands down. All sin can do is threaten us with death.... Grace...invites us into life—a life that goes on and on and on, world without end.

ROMANS 5:20–21 MSG

I am the Light of the world; he who follows Me will not walk in the darkness, but will have the Light of life.

JOHN 8:12 NASB

We're not giving up. How could we! Even though on the outside it often looks like things are falling apart on us, on the inside, where God is making new life, not a day goes by without his unfolding grace.

2 CORINTHIANS 4:16 MSG

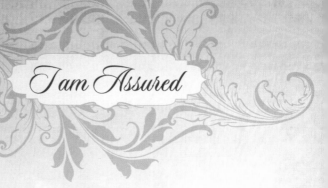

# I am Assured

Your promises have been thoroughly tested,
and your servant loves them.
…My eyes stay open through the watches of the night,
that I may meditate on your promises.

Psalm 119:140, 148 niv

He has granted to us his precious and very great promises,
so that through them you may become partakers of the
divine nature, having escaped from the corruption that is
in the world.

2 Peter 1:3-4 esv

To him who is able to do immeasurably more than all
we ask or imagine, according to his power that is at work
within us, to him be glory…for ever and ever! Amen.

Ephesians 3:20–21 niv

All of God's promises have been fulfilled in Christ
with a resounding "Yes!"

2 Corinthians 1:20 nlt

These things I have written to you who believe in the
name of the Son of God, that you may know that you
have eternal life, and that you may continue to believe in
the name of the Son of God.

1 John 5:13 nkjv

Jesus Christ is the same yesterday and today and forever.

Hebrews 13:8 nasb

The Lord always keeps his promises;
he is gracious in all he does.

Psalm 145:13 nlt

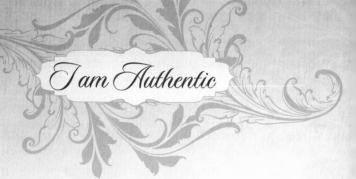

# I am Authentic

If you're content to simply be yourself,
your life will count for plenty.

MATTHEW 23:12 MSG

It's who you are and the way you live that count before
God. Your worship must engage your spirit in the pursuit
of truth. That's the kind of people the Father is out
looking for: those who are simply and honestly *themselves*
before him in their worship. God is sheer being itself—
Spirit. Those who worship him must do it out of their
very being, their spirits, their true selves, in adoration.

JOHN 4:23–24 MSG

Take your everyday, ordinary life—your sleeping, eating, going-to-work, and walking-around life—and place it before God as an offering. Embracing what God does for you is the best thing you can do for him. Don't become so well-adjusted to your culture that you fit into it without even thinking. Instead, fix your attention on God. You'll be changed from the inside out. Readily recognize what he wants from you, and quickly respond to it. Unlike the culture around you, always dragging you down to its level of immaturity, God brings the best out of you, develops well-formed maturity in you.

Romans 12:1–2 MSG

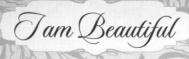

## I am Beautiful

I will praise You,
for I am fearfully and wonderfully made;
Marvelous are Your works,
And that my soul knows very well.

Psalm 139:14 NKJV

Don't be concerned about the outward beauty of fancy
hairstyles, expensive jewelry, or beautiful clothes. You
should clothe yourselves instead with the beauty that
comes from within, the unfading beauty of a gentle and
quiet spirit, which is so precious to God.

1 Peter 3:3–4 NLT

The LORD doesn't see things the way you see them.
People judge by outward appearance,
but the LORD looks at the heart.

1 SAMUEL 16:7 NLT

Has anyone by fussing in front of the mirror ever gotten taller by so much as an inch? All this time and money wasted on fashion—do you think it makes that much difference? Instead of looking at the fashions, walk out into the fields and look at the wildflowers. They never primp or shop, but have you ever seen color and design quite like it? The ten best-dressed men and women in the country look shabby alongside them.

MATTHEW 6:27–29 MSG

He has made everything beautiful in its time.

ECCLESIASTES 3:11 NIV

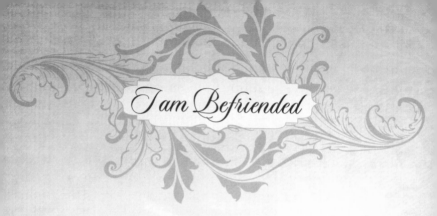

# I am Befriended

The LORD is near to all who call on him,
to all who call on him in truth.

PSALM 145:18 NIV

Here I am! I stand at the door and knock. If anyone hears
my voice and opens the door, I will come in and eat with
that person, and they with me.

REVELATION 3:20 NIV

Turn to me and have mercy,
for I am alone and in deep distress.

PSALM 25:16 NLT

The amazing grace of the Master, Jesus Christ, the
extravagant love of God, the intimate friendship of the

Holy Spirit, be with all of you.

2 Corinthians 13:14 msg

The right word at the right time
is like a custom-made piece of jewelry,
And a wise friend's timely reprimand
is like a gold ring slipped on your finger.
Reliable friends who do what they say
are like cool drinks in sweltering heat—refreshing!

Proverbs 25:12–13 msg

By this we know that we abide in Him and He in us,
because He has given us of His Spirit.

1 John 4:13 nasb

A friend loves at all times.

Proverbs 17:17 nkjv

Behold, I am with you always, to the end of the age.

Matthew 28:20 esv

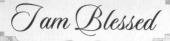
*I am Blessed*

You prepare a feast for me
in the presence of my enemies.
You honor me by anointing my head with oil.
My cup overflows with blessings.

Psalm 23:5 nlt

Blessed be the God and Father of our Lord Jesus Christ,
who has blessed us in Christ with every spiritual blessing
in the heavenly places, even as he chose us in him before
the foundation of the world, that we should be holy and
blameless before him.

Ephesians 1:3–4 esv

How blessed all those in whom you live,

whose lives become roads you travel;

They wind through lonesome valleys, come upon brooks,

discover cool springs and pools brimming with rain!

PSALM 84:5–6 MSG

From his abundance we have all received one gracious

blessing after another.

JOHN 1:16 NLT

For the LORD God is our sun and our shield.

He gives us grace and glory.

The LORD will withhold no good thing

from those who do what is right.

PSALM 84:11 NLT

The LORD bless you, and keep you;

The LORD make His face shine on you,

And be gracious to you;

The LORD lift up His countenance on you,

And give you peace.

NUMBERS 6:24–26 NASB

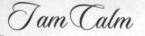
*I am Calm*

Be still in the presence of the LORD,

and wait patiently for him to act.

Don't worry about evil people who prosper

or fret about their wicked schemes.

Stop being angry!

Turn from your rage!

Do not lose your temper—

it only leads to harm.

PSALM 37:7-8 NLT

Let not your heart be troubled.

You are trusting God, now trust in me.

JOHN 14:1 TLB

Cast all your anxiety on him because he cares for you.

1 PETER 5:7 NIV

Be still, and know that I am God.
I will be exalted among the nations,
I will be exalted in the earth!

Psalm 46:10 esv

Do not be anxious about anything, but in every situation,
by prayer and petition, with thanksgiving, present
your requests to God.

Philippians 4:6 niv

In my trouble I cried to the Lord,
And He answered me.

Psalm 120:1 nasb

I want you woven into a tapestry of love, in touch with
everything there is to know of God. Then you will have
minds confident and at rest, focused on Christ,
God's great mystery.

Colossians 2:2 msg

Trusting me, you will be unshakable and assured, deeply at
peace. In this godless world you will continue to experience
difficulties. But take heart! I've conquered the world.

John 16:33 msg

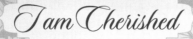

# I am Cherished

The Lord directs the steps of the godly.
He delights in every detail of their lives.
Though they stumble, they will never fall,
for the Lord holds them by the hand.

Psalm 37:23–24 NLT

I am sure that neither death nor life, nor angels nor rulers,
nor things present nor things to come, nor powers, nor height
nor depth, nor anything else in all creation, will be able to
separate us from the love of God in Christ Jesus our Lord.

Romans 8:38–39 ESV

He tends his flock like a shepherd:

He gathers the lambs in his arms

and carries them close to his heart;

he gently leads those that have young.

ISAIAH 40:11 NIV


Blessed be the LORD,

Because He has heard the voice of my supplication.

The LORD is my strength and my shield;

My heart trusts in Him, and I am helped;

Therefore my heart exults,

And with my song I shall thank Him.

PSALM 28:6-7 NASB


You're blessed when you feel you've lost what is

most dear to you. Only then can you be embraced

by the One most dear to you.

MATTHEW 5:4 MSG

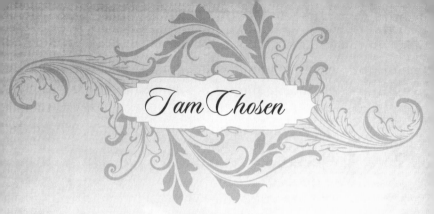

# *I am Chosen*

How blessed is God!... Long before he laid down earth's
foundations, he had us in mind, had settled on us as the
focus of his love, to be made whole and holy by his love.
Long, long ago he decided to adopt us into his family
through Jesus Christ. (What pleasure he took in planning
this!) He wanted us to enter into the celebration of his
lavish gift-giving by the hand of his beloved Son.

EPHESIANS 1:3–6 MSG

We know that all things work together for good
to those who love God, to those who are the called
according to His purpose.

ROMANS 8:28 NKJV

Confirm God's invitation to you, his choice of you.
Don't put it off; do it now. Do this, and you'll have
your life on a firm footing.

2 PETER 1:10–11 MSG

There is a time for everything,
and everything on earth has its special season.

ECCLESIASTES 3:1 NCV

No eye has seen, no ear has heard,
and no mind has imagined
what God has prepared
for those who love him.

1 CORINTHIANS 2:9 NLT

You are a chosen people, a royal priesthood, a holy nation,
God's special possession, that you may declare the praises of
him who called you out of darkness into his wonderful light.

1 PETER 2:9 NIV

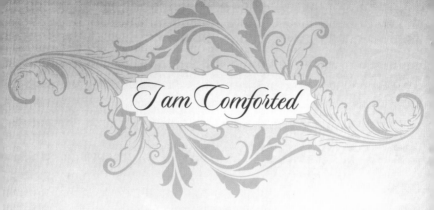

# I am Comforted

To all who mourn...he will give: beauty for ashes;
joy instead of mourning; praise instead of heaviness.
For God has planted them like strong and
graceful oaks for his own glory.

ISAIAH 61:3 TLB

May your unfailing love be my comfort,
according to your promise to your servant.

PSALM 119:76 NIV

May our Lord Jesus Christ himself and God our Father,
who loved us and by his grace gave us eternal comfort and
a wonderful hope, comfort you and strengthen you.

2 THESSALONIANS 2:16–17 NLT

Unless the LORD had helped me,

I would soon have settled in the silence of the grave.

I cried out, "I am slipping!"

but your unfailing love, O LORD, supported me.

When doubts filled my mind,

your comfort gave me renewed hope and cheer.

PSALM 94:17–19 NLT


Praise be to the God and Father of our Lord Jesus Christ,

the Father of compassion and the God of all comfort.

2 CORINTHIANS 1:3 NIV


God's dwelling place is now among the people, and he will

dwell with them…. "He will wipe every tear from their

eyes. There will be no more death" or mourning or crying

or pain, for the old order of things has passed away.

REVELATION 21:3–4 NIV

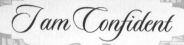

# I am Confident

Be my rock of refuge,

to which I can always go;

give the command to save me,

for you are my rock and my fortress....

You have been my hope, Sovereign LORD,

my confidence since my youth.

PSALM 71:3, 5 NIV

This is the confidence that we have toward him, that if we
ask anything according to his will he hears us. And if we
know that he hears us in whatever we ask, we know that
we have the requests that we have asked of him.

1 JOHN 5:14–15 ESV

Let us then approach God's throne of grace with confidence, so that we may receive mercy and find grace to help us in our time of need.

We can confidently say, "The Lord is my helper; I will not fear; what can man do to me?"

HEBREWS 13:6 ESV

I am confident of this very thing, that He who began a good work in you will perfect it until the day of Christ Jesus.

PHILIPPIANS 1:6 NASB

But if you remain in me and my words remain in you, you may ask for anything you want, and it will be granted!

JOHN 15:7 NLT

I can do everything through Christ, who gives me strength.

PHILIPPIANS 4:13 NLT

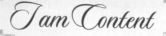

# I am Content

Oh, how sweet the light of day,
and how wonderful to live in the sunshine!
Even if you live a long time,
don't take a single day for granted.
Take delight in each light-filled hour.

ECCLESIASTES 11:7–8 MSG

I know what it is to be in need, and I know what it is to
have plenty. I have learned the secret of being content
in any and every situation, whether well fed or hungry,
whether living in plenty or in want. I can do all this
through him who gives me strength.

PHILIPPIANS 4:12-13 NIV

If God cares so wonderfully for wildflowers that are here
today and thrown into the fire tomorrow, he will certainly
care for you. Why do you have so little faith? So don't
worry about these things, saying, "What will we eat?
What will we drink? What will we wear?" These things
dominate the thoughts of unbelievers, but your heavenly
Father already knows all your needs. Seek the Kingdom
of God above all else, and live righteously, and he will give
you everything you need.

Matthew 6:30-33 nlt

You're blessed when you're content with just who you are—
no more, no less. That's the moment you find yourselves
proud owners of everything that can't be bought.

Matthew 5:5 msg

# I am Courageous

Love the LORD, all you godly ones!
For the LORD protects those who are loyal to him,
but he harshly punishes the arrogant.
So be strong and courageous,
all you who put your hope in the LORD!

PSALM 31:23–24 NLT

May he give you the power to accomplish all the good
things your faith prompts you to do.

2 THESSALONIANS 1:11 NLT

Be strong and courageous. Do not be frightened,
and do not be dismayed, for the LORD your God
is with you wherever you go.

JOSHUA 1:9 ESV

Even though I walk through the valley of the shadow of death,
I fear no evil, for You are with me;
Your rod and Your staff, they comfort me.

PSALM 23:4 NASB

I eagerly expect and hope that I will in no way be
ashamed, but will have sufficient courage so that
now as always Christ will be exalted in my body,
whether by life or by death.

PHILIPPIANS 1:20 NIV

When I am afraid, I put my trust in you.
In God, whose word I praise—
in God I trust and am not afraid.

PSALM 56:3–4 NIV

Be on guard. Stand firm in the faith. Be courageous.
Be strong. And do everything with love.

1 CORINTHIANS 16:13–14 NLT

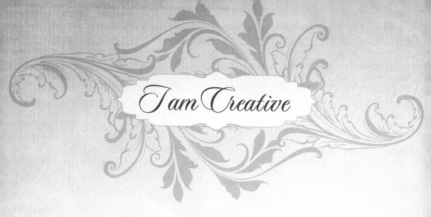

# I am Creative

Having then gifts differing according to the grace that is given to us, let us use them.

ROMANS 12:6 NKJV

The heavens are telling of the glory of God;
And their expanse is declaring the work of His hands.

PSALM 19:1 NASB

O LORD, what a variety of things you have made!
In wisdom you have made them all.
The earth is full of your creatures.

PSALM 104:24 NLT

Be sure to use the abilities God has given you.

1 TIMOTHY 4:14 TLB

The LORD is the one who shaped the mountains,
stirs up the winds, and reveals his thoughts to mankind.
He turns the light of dawn into darkness
and treads on the heights of the earth.
The LORD God of Heaven's Armies is his name!

AMOS 4:13 NLT

He has filled him with divine spirit, with skill, intelligence,
and knowledge in every kind of craft.

EXODUS 35:31 NRSV

Let the beauty of the LORD our God be upon us,
And establish the work of our hands for us.

PSALM 90:17 NKJV

A man's gift makes room for him
And brings him before great men.

PROVERBS 18:16 NASB

Do you see people skilled in their work?
They will work for kings, not for ordinary people.

PROVERBS 22:29 NCV

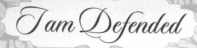

# I am Defended

Beloved, do not avenge yourselves, but rather give place to wrath; for it is written, "Vengeance is Mine, I will repay," says the Lord.

ROMANS 12:19 NKJV

He will not break the bruised reed, nor quench the dimly burning flame. He will encourage the fainthearted, those tempted to despair. He will see full justice given to all who have been wronged.

ISAIAH 42:3 TLB

The LORD secures justice for the poor
and upholds the cause of the needy.

PSALM 140:12 NIV

He will not judge by appearance, false evidence,

or hearsay, but will defend the poor and the exploited.

He will rule against the wicked who oppress them. For he

will be clothed with fairness and with truth.

ISAIAH 11:3–5 TLB

He did not retaliate when he was insulted,

nor threaten revenge when he suffered.

He left his case in the hands of God,

who always judges fairly.

1 PETER 2:23 NLT

LORD, you know the hopes of the helpless.

Surely you will hear their cries and comfort them.

You will bring justice to the orphans and the oppressed,

so mere people can no longer terrify them.

PSALM 10:17–18 NLT

Righteousness and justice

are the foundation of Your throne.

PSALM 89:14 NKJV

# *I am Delivered*

I waited patiently for the LORD;

he turned to me and heard my cry.

He lifted me out of the slimy pit,

out of the mud and mire;

he set my feet on a rock

and gave me a firm place to stand.

He put a new song in my mouth,

a hymn of praise to our God.

Many will see and fear the LORD;

and put their trust in him.

PSALM 40:1–3 NIV


The LORD hears his people when they call to him for help.

He rescues them from all their troubles.

PSALM 34:17 NLT

Humble yourselves in the sight of the Lord,
and He will lift you up.

JAMES 4:10 NKJV

The righteous person faces many troubles,
but the LORD comes to the rescue each time.

PSALM 34:19 NLT

My prayer is to you, O LORD.
At an acceptable time, O God,
in the abundance of your steadfast love answer me in your
saving faithfulness.
Deliver me
from sinking in the mire;
let me be delivered from my enemies
and from the deep waters.
Answer me, O LORD , for your steadfast love is good;
according to your abundant mercy, turn to me.

PSALM 69:13-14, 16 ESV

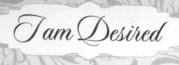
*I am Desired*

I am my beloved's,
And his desire is toward me.

Song of Solomon 7:10 NKJV

It's in Christ that we find out who we are and what we
are living for. Long before we first heard of Christ and got
our hopes up, he had his eye on us, had designs on us for
glorious living, part of the overall purpose he is working
out in everything and everyone.

Ephesians 1:11–12 MSG

You make known to me the path of life;
you will fill me with joy in your presence,
with eternal pleasures at your right hand.

Psalm 16:11 NIV

The LORD your God is living among you.

He is a mighty savior.

He will take delight in you with gladness.

With his love, he will calm all your fears.

He will rejoice over you with joyful songs.

ZEPHANIAH 3:17 NLT


My God is changeless in his love for me,

and he will come and help me.

PSALM 59:10 TLB


My beloved speaks and says to me:

"Arise, my love, my beautiful one,

and come away,

for behold, the winter is past;

the rain is over and gone.

The flowers appear on the earth,

the time of singing has come."

SONG OF SOLOMON 2:10-12 ESV

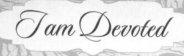

# I am Devoted

With all my heart I have sought You;
Do not let me wander from Your commandments.
Your word I have treasured in my heart,
That I may not sin against You.
…Teach me, O Lord, the way of Your statutes,
And I shall observe it to the end.

PSALM 119:10–11, 33 NASB

Seek first the kingdom of God and His righteousness, and
all these things shall be added to you.

MATTHEW 6:33 NKJV

Commit everything you do to the Lord.
Trust him, and he will help you.

PSALM 37:5 NLT

Stand firm. Let nothing move you. Always give yourselves fully to the work of the Lord, because you know that your labor in the Lord is not in vain.

1 CORINTHIANS 15:58 NIV

Commit your work to the LORD,
and your plans will be established.

PROVERBS 16:3 ESV

May God himself, the God of peace, sanctify you through and through. May your whole spirit, soul and body be kept blameless at the coming of our Lord Jesus Christ. The one who calls you is faithful, and he will do it.

1 THESSALONIANS 5:23–24 NIV

If any of you wants to be my follower, you must turn from your selfish ways, take up your cross daily, and follow me.

LUKE 9:23 NLT

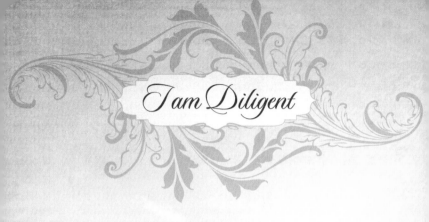

# I am Diligent

The plans of the diligent lead to profit
as surely as haste leads to poverty.

PROVERBS 21:5 NIV

To enjoy your work and to accept your lot in life—
that is indeed a gift from God. The person who does that
will not need to look back with sorrow on his past,
for God gives him joy.

ECCLESIASTES 5:20 TLB

In all the work you are doing, work the best you can.
Work as if you were doing it for the Lord, not for people.

COLOSSIANS 3:23 NCV

Be diligent in these matters; give yourself wholly to them,
so that everyone may see your progress.

1 TIMOTHY 4:15 NIV


Wise words bring many benefits,
and hard work brings rewards.

PROVERBS 12:14 NLT


Finish the work, so that your eager willingness to do it
may be matched by your completion of it,
according to your means.

2 CORINTHIANS 8:11 NIV


Pay careful attention to your own work,
for then you will get the satisfaction of a job well done,
and you won't need to compare yourself to anyone else.
For we are each responsible for our own conduct.

GALATIANS 6:4–5 NLT

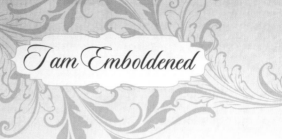

# I am Emboldened

We are pressed on every side by troubles, but we are not crushed. We are perplexed, but not driven to despair. We are hunted down, but never abandoned by God. We get knocked down, but we are not destroyed.

2 Corinthians 4:8–9 nlt

If you're serious about living this new resurrection life with Christ, *act* like it. Pursue the things over which Christ presides. Don't shuffle along, eyes to the ground, absorbed with the things right in front of you. Look up, and be alert to what is going on around Christ—that's where the action is. See things from *his* perspective.

Colossians 3:1–2 msg

Let us therefore come boldly to the throne of grace,

that we may obtain mercy and find grace

to help in time of need.

HEBREWS 4:16 NKJV

In all this you greatly rejoice, though now for a little while
you may have had to suffer grief in all kinds of trials.
These have come so that the proven genuineness of your
faith—of greater worth than gold, which perishes even
though refined by fire—may result in praise, glory and
honor when Jesus Christ is revealed.

1 PETER 1:6–7 NIV

# I am Encouraged

Though an army besiege me,
my heart will not fear;
though war break out against me,
even then I will be confident.
One thing I ask from the LORD,
this only do I seek:
that I may dwell in the house of the LORD
all the days of my life,
to gaze on the beauty of the LORD
and to seek him in his temple.
For in the day of trouble
he will keep me safe in his dwelling.

PSALM 27:3-5 NIV

The humble will see their God at work and be glad.
Let all who seek God's help be encouraged.

PSALM 69:32 NLT

May the God who gives endurance and
encouragement give you the same attitude of mind
toward each other that Christ Jesus had.

ROMANS 15:5 NIV

We do not lose heart, but though our outer man is
decaying, yet our inner man is being renewed day by day.
For momentary, light affliction is producing for us an
eternal weight of glory far beyond all comparison.

2 CORINTHIANS 4:16–17 NASB

Let us consider how to stir up one another to love and
good works, not neglecting to meet together, as is the
habit of some, but encouraging one another.

HEBREWS 10:24–25 ESV

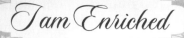

# I am Enriched

God's blessing makes life rich;
nothing we do can improve on God.

PROVERBS 10:22 MSG

Oh, the depth of the riches both of the wisdom
and knowledge of God! How unsearchable are
His judgments and unfathomable His ways!

ROMANS 11:33 NASB

Every good gift and every perfect gift is from above,
coming down from the Father of lights with whom
there is no variation or shadow due to change.

JAMES 1:17 ESV

Everything God created is good, and nothing is to be
rejected if it is received with thanksgiving.

1 TIMOTHY 4:4 NIV

I will tell of the kindnesses of the LORD,

the deeds for which he is to be praised,

according to all the LORD has done for us...

according to his compassion and many kindnesses.

ISAIAH 63:7 NIV

A good man's speech reveals the rich treasures within him.

MATTHEW 12:35 TLB

Blessed are those who find wisdom,

those who gain understanding,

for she is more profitable than silver

and yields better returns than gold.

She is more precious than rubies;

nothing you desire can compare with her.

Long life is in her right hand;

in her left hand are riches and honor.

Her ways are pleasant ways,

and all her paths are peace.

PROVERBS 3:13–17 NIV

# I am Enthusiastic

Work with enthusiasm, as though you were working
for the Lord rather than for people.

EPHESIANS 6:7 NLT

We should make the most of what God gives,
both the bounty and the capacity to enjoy it, accepting
what's given and delighting in the work. It's God's gift!

ECCLESIASTES 5:19 MSG

By You I can run against a troop,
By my God I can leap over a wall.

PSALM 18:29 NKJV

Whatever your hand finds to do, do it with all your might.

ECCLESIASTES 9:10 NIV

Everything else is worthless when compared with the
priceless gain of knowing Christ Jesus my Lord.
I have put aside all else, counting it worth less than
nothing, in order that I can have Christ.... Now I have
given up everything else—I have found it to be the only
way to really know Christ and to experience the mighty
power that brought him back to life again, and to find out
what it means to suffer and to die with him. So whatever
it takes, I will be one who lives in the fresh newness of life
of those who are alive from the dead.

PHILIPPIANS 3:8,10-11 TLB

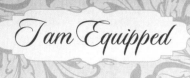

# I am Equipped

All scripture is inspired by God and is useful for
teaching, for reproof, for correction, and for training in
righteousness, so that everyone who belongs to God may
be proficient, equipped for every good work.

2 TIMOTHY 3:16–17 NRSV

May He give you the power to accomplish all
the good things your faith prompts you to do.

2 THESSALONIANS 1:11 NLT

Then the LORD reached out his hand and touched
my mouth and said to me, "I have put my words
in your mouth."

JEREMIAH 1:9 NIV

We are God's handiwork, created in Christ Jesus to do
good works, which God prepared in advance for us to do.

Ephesians 2:10 niv

So then, my beloved, just as you have always obeyed,
not as in my presence only, but now much more in my
absence, work out your salvation with fear and trembling;
for it is God who is at work in you, both to will and to
work for His good pleasure.

Philippians 2:12-13 nasb

If any of you lacks wisdom, you should ask God,
who gives generously to all without finding fault,
and it will be given to you.

James 1:5 niv

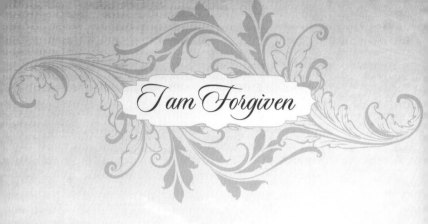

# I am Forgiven

For You, Lord, are good, and ready to forgive,
And abundant in mercy to all those who call upon You.

PSALM 86:5 NKJV

Whenever you stand praying, forgive, if you have anything
against anyone, so that your Father also who is in heaven
may forgive you.

MARK 11:25 ESV

As far as the east is from the west,
So far has He removed our transgressions from us.

PSALM 103:12 NASB

If we confess our sins, He is faithful and just to forgive us
our sins and to cleanse us from all unrighteousness.

1 John 1:9 nkjv

He is so rich in kindness and grace that he purchased our
freedom with the blood of his Son and forgave our sins.

Ephesians 1:7 nlt

My sacrifice, O God, is a broken spirit;
a broken and contrite heart
you, God, will not despise.

Psalm 51:17 niv

Her sins—and they are many—have been forgiven,
so she has shown me much love. But a person who
is forgiven little shows only little love.

Luke 7:47 nlt

If you forgive other people when they sin against you,
your heavenly Father will also forgive you.

Matthew 6:14 niv

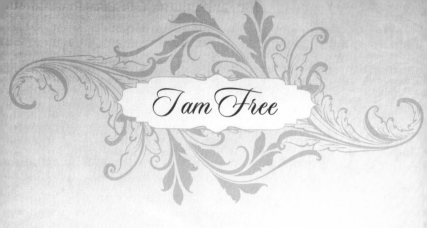

# I am Free

Now that you have been set free from sin and have
become slaves of God, the benefit you reap leads to
holiness, and the result is eternal life.

Romans 6:22 niv

Jesus said, "If you hold to my teaching,
you are really my disciples. Then you will know the truth,
and the truth will set you free."

John 8:31–32 niv

So Christ has truly set us free. Now make sure that you
stay free, and don't get tied up again in slavery to the law.

Galatians 5:1 nlt

He has delivered us from the power of darkness and
conveyed us into the kingdom of the Son of His love.

COLOSSIANS 1:13 NKJV

There is now no condemnation for those who are in
Christ Jesus, because through Christ Jesus
the law of the Spirit who gives life has
set you free from the law of sin and death.

ROMANS 8:1–2 NIV

Understand what we are telling you: You can have
forgiveness of your sins through Jesus. The law of Moses
could not free you from your sins. But through Jesus
everyone who believes is free from all sins.

ACTS 13:38-39 NCV

Now the Lord is the Spirit, and where
the Spirit of the Lord is, there is freedom.

2 CORINTHIANS 3:17 NRSV

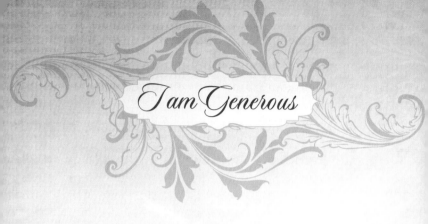

# I am Generous

Let each one give as he purposes in his heart, not grudgingly or of necessity; for God loves a cheerful giver.

2 CORINTHIANS 9:7 NKJV

It is more blessed to give than to receive.

ACTS 20:35 NIV

One man gives freely, yet gains even more;
another withholds unduly, but comes to poverty.
A generous man will prosper;
whoever refreshes others will be refreshed.

PROVERBS 11:24–25 NIV

Whoever is generous to the poor lends to the Lord,
and he will repay him for his deed.

PROVERBS 19:17 ESV

When you give to the needy, do not let your left hand
know what your right hand is doing, so that
your giving may be in secret. Then your Father,
who sees what is done in secret, will reward you.

MATTHEW 6:3–4 NIV

You shall generously give to him, and your heart
shall not be grieved when you give to him,
because for this thing the Lord your God will bless you
in all your work and in all your undertakings.

DEUTERONOMY 15:10 NASB

The generous will themselves be blessed,
for they share their food with the poor.

PROVERBS 22:9 NIV

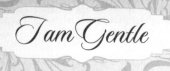

# I am Gentle

A gentle answer deflects anger,
but harsh words make tempers flare.

PROVERBS 15:1 NLT

In your hearts revere Christ as Lord.
Always be prepared to give an answer to everyone who
asks you to give the reason for the hope that you have.
But do this with gentleness and respect.

1 PETER 3:15 NIV

Remind the believers to yield to the authority of rulers
and government leaders, to obey them, to be ready to
do good, to speak no evil about anyone, to live in peace,
and to be gentle and polite to all people.

TITUS 3:1-2 NCV

The wisdom that comes from heaven is first of all pure
and full of quiet gentleness. Then it is peace-loving
and courteous. It allows discussion and is willing
to yield to others; it is full of mercy and good deeds.
It is wholehearted and straightforward and sincere.

JAMES 3:17 TLB


Blessed are the gentle, for they shall inherit the earth.

MATTHEW 5:5 NASB


Let your gentleness be evident to all. The Lord is near.

PHILIPPIANS 4:5 NIV


You have given me the shield of your salvation,
and your right hand supported me,
and your gentleness made me great.

PSALM 18:35 ESV

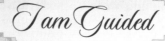

# I am Guided

Whether you turn to the right or to the left,
your ears will hear a voice behind you, saying,
"This is the way; walk in it."

ISAIAH 30:21 NIV


We can make our plans,
but the LORD determines our steps.

PROVERBS 16:9 NLT


Guide me in your truth and teach me,
for you are God my Savior,
and my hope is in you all day long.

PSALM 25:5 NIV

The true children of God are those who let
God's Spirit lead them.

ROMANS 8:14 NCV

Trust in the LORD with all your heart,
And lean not on your own understanding;
In all your ways acknowledge Him,
And He shall direct your paths.

PROVERBS 3:5–6 NKJV

We ask God to give you complete knowledge of his will
and to give you spiritual wisdom and understanding.
Then the way you live will always honor and please the
Lord, and your lives will produce every kind of good fruit.
All the while, you will grow as you learn to know
God better and better.

COLOSSIANS 1:9–10 NLT

Listen to advice and accept discipline,
and at the end you will be counted among the wise.

PROVERBS 19:20 NIV

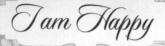
*I am Happy*

Happy are those who hear the joyful call to worship,
for they will walk in the light of your presence, Lord.

Psalm 89:15 nlt

May you be filled with joy, always thanking the Father. He
has enabled you to share in the inheritance that belongs to
his people, who live in the light.

Colossians 1:11–12 nlt

Enter his gates with thanksgiving,
and his courts with praise.
Give thanks to him, bless his name.
For the Lord is good;
his steadfast love endures forever,
and his faithfulness to all generations.

Psalm 100:4–5 nrsv

He will yet fill your mouth with laughter
and your lips with shouts of joy.

JOB 8:21 NIV

The Lord has done great things for us,
and we are filled with joy.

PSALM 126:3 NIV

I know that there is nothing better for people than to be
happy and to do good while they live.

ECCLESIASTES 3:12 NIV

I will give thanks to the LORD with my whole heart;
I will recount all of your wonderful deeds.
I will be glad and exult in you;
I will sing praise to your name, O Most High.

PSALM 9:1-2 ESV

Rejoice in the Lord always. Again I will say, rejoice!

PHILIPPIANS 4:4 NKJV

# I am Healed

Trust God from the bottom of your heart;

don't try to figure out everything on your own.

Listen for God's voice in everything you do,

everywhere you go;

he's the one who will keep you on track.

Don't assume that you know it all.

Run to God! Run from evil!

Your body will glow with health,

your very bones will vibrate with life!

PROVERBS 3:5–8 MSG


He was pierced for our transgressions,

he was crushed for our iniquities;

the punishment that brought us peace was on him,

and by his wounds we are healed.

ISAIAH 53:5 NIV

A cheerful heart does good like medicine.

PROVERBS 17:22 TLB

Daughter, your faith has made you well;
go in peace and be healed of your affliction.

MARK 5:34 NASB

My child, pay attention to what I say.
Listen carefully to my words.
Don't lose sight of them.
Let them penetrate deep into your heart,
for they bring life to those who find them,
and healing to their whole body.

PROVERBS 4:20–22 NLT

The world and its desires pass away,
but whoever does the will of God lives forever.

1 JOHN 2:17 NIV

# *I am Heaven-bound*

We fix our eyes not on what is seen,
but on what is unseen, since what is seen is temporary,
but what is unseen is eternal.

2 Corinthians 4:18 niv

Before the mountains were brought forth,
or ever you had formed the earth and the world,
from everlasting to everlasting you are God.

Psalm 90:2 esv

Surely goodness and mercy shall follow me
All the days of my life;
And I will dwell in the house of the Lord
Forever.

Psalm 23:6 nkjv

We are citizens of heaven, where the Lord Jesus Christ lives.
And we are eagerly waiting for him to return as our Savior.
He will take our weak mortal bodies and change them into
glorious bodies like his own, using the same power with
which he will bring everything under his control.

PHILIPPIANS 3:20–21 NLT

I'm asking GOD for one thing,
only one thing:
To live with him in his house
my whole life long.
I'll contemplate his beauty;
I'll study at his feet.

PSALM 27:4 MSG

I will come back and take you to be with me that you also
may be where I am.

JOHN 14:3 NIV

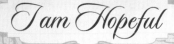

# I am Hopeful

GOD...rekindles burned-out lives with fresh hope,

Restoring dignity and respect to their lives—

a place in the sun!

1 SAMUEL 2:7–8 MSG

Blessed be the God and Father of our Lord Jesus Christ!

According to his great mercy, he has caused us to be born

again to a living hope through the resurrection of Jesus Christ.

1 PETER 1:3 ESV

The LORD is good to those whose hope is in him,

to the one who seeks him.

LAMENTATIONS 3:25 NIV

There is surely a future hope for you,
and your hope will not be cut off.

PROVERBS 23:18 NIV

We can rejoice, too, when we run into problems and trials,
for we know that they help us develop endurance. And
endurance develops strength of character, and character
strengthens our confident hope of salvation. And this
hope will not lead to disappointment. For we know how
dearly God loves us, because he has given us the Holy
Spirit to fill our hearts with his love.

ROMANS 5:3–5 NLT

May the God of hope fill you with all joy and
peace as you trust in him, so that you may overflow
with hope by the power of the Holy Spirit.

ROMANS 15:13 NIV

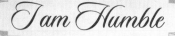

# I am Humble

Humility is the fear of the LORD;
its wages are riches and honor and life.

PROVERBS 22:4 NIV

Where you have envy and selfish ambition, there you
find disorder and every evil practice. But the wisdom that
comes from heaven is first of all pure; then peace-loving,
considerate, submissive, full of mercy and good fruit,
impartial and sincere. Peacemakers who sow in peace reap
a harvest of righteousness.

JAMES 3:16–18 NIV

Those who accept correction gain understanding.

Respect for the LORD will teach you wisdom.

If you want to be honored, you must be humble.

PROVERBS 15:32–33 NCV

In your relationships with one another, have the same

mindset as Christ Jesus:

Who, being in very nature God,

did not consider equality with God something

to be used to his own advantage;

rather, he made himself nothing

by taking the very nature of a servant,

being made in human likeness.

And being found in appearance as a man,

he humbled himself

by becoming obedient to death—

even death on a cross!

Therefore God exalted him to the highest place

and gave him the name that is above every name.

PHILIPPIANS 2:5–9 NIV

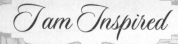

## I am Inspired

The precepts of the LORD are right,

giving joy to the heart.

The commands of the LORD are radiant,

giving light to the eyes.

PSALM 19:8 NIV

I am the Light of the world; he who follows Me will not

walk in the darkness, but will have the Light of life.

JOHN 8:12 NASB

Your laws are my treasure; they are my heart's delight.

PSALM 119:111 NLT

Pursue a righteous life—a life of wonder, faith, love, steadiness, courtesy. Run hard and fast in the faith. Seize the eternal life, the life you were called to, the life you so fervently embraced in the presence of so many witnesses.

1 Timothy 6:11–12 msg

I have been crucified with Christ;
and it is no longer I who live,
but Christ lives in me.

Galatians 2:20 nasb

You are the light of the world. A city set on a hill
cannot be hidden. Nor do people light a lamp
and put it under a basket, but on a stand,
and it gives light to all in the house. In the same way,
let your light shine before others, so that they may
see your good works and give glory to your
Father who is in heaven.

Matthew 5:14–16 esv

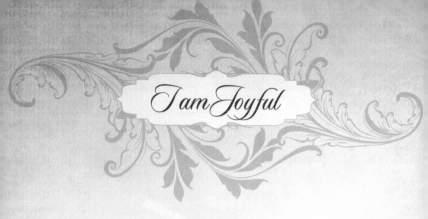

# I am Joyful

Satisfy us in the morning with your unfailing love,
that we may sing for joy and be glad all our days.

Psalm 90:14 niv

Be truly glad. There is wonderful joy ahead....
You love him even though you have never seen him.
Though you do not see him now, you trust him;
and you rejoice with a glorious, inexpressible joy.

1 Peter 1:6, 8 nlt

Until now you have not asked for anything in my name.
Ask and you will receive, and your joy will be complete.

John 16:24 niv

Let all those rejoice who put their trust in You;

Let them ever shout for joy, because You defend them;

Let those also who love Your name

Be joyful in You.

PSALM 5:11 NKJV

Our mouth was filled with laughter,

and our tongue with shouts of joy.

PSALM 126:2 ESV

I have told you this so that my joy may be in you

and that your joy may be complete.

JOHN 15:11 NIV

You will go out in joy

and be led forth in peace;

the mountains and hills

will burst into song before you,

and all the trees of the field

will clap their hands.

ISAIAH 55:12 NIV

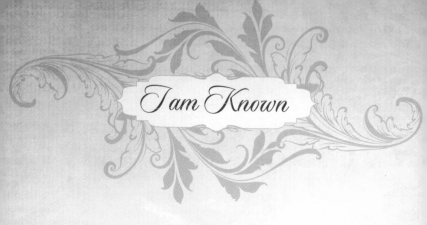

# I am Known

God's solid foundation stands firm, sealed with this inscription: "The Lord knows those who are his."

2 TIMOTHY 2:19 NIV

When I was a child, I spoke and thought and reasoned as a child. But when I grew up, I put away childish things. Now we see things imperfectly, like puzzling reflections in a mirror, but then we will see everything with perfect clarity. All that I know now is partial and incomplete, but then I will know everything completely, just as God now knows me completely.

1 CORINTHIANS 13:11-12 NLT

"For I know the plans I have for you," declares the Lord,

"plans to prosper you and not to harm you,

plans to give you hope and a future."

Jeremiah 29:11 niv

I will instruct you and teach you in the way you should go;

I will counsel you with my loving eye on you.

Psalm 32:8 niv

O Lord, You have searched me and known me.

You know my sitting down and my rising up;

You understand my thought afar off.

You comprehend my path and my lying down,

And are acquainted with all my ways.

For there is not a word on my tongue,

But behold, Lord, You know it altogether.

Psalm 139:1–4 nkjv

# I am Loved

The steadfast love of the LORD never ceases;

his mercies never come to an end;

they are new every morning;

great is your faithfulness.

LAMENTATIONS 3:22–23 ESV


Know therefore that the LORD your God is God;

he is the faithful God, keeping his covenant of love

to a thousand generations of those who love him

and keep his commandments.

DEUTERONOMY 7:9 NIV


Let love and faithfulness never leave you;

bind them around your neck,

write them on the tablet of your heart.

PROVERBS 3:3 NIV

We have come to know and have believed the love
which God has for us. God is love, and the one who
abides in love abides in God, and God abides in him.
We love, because He first loved us.

1 John 4:16, 19 nasb


You, O Lord, are good and forgiving,
abounding in steadfast love to all who call upon you.

Psalm 86:5 esv


Three things will last forever—faith, hope, and love—
and the greatest of these is love.

1 Corinthians 13:13 nlt


I will sing of the Lord's great love forever;
with my mouth I will make your faithfulness known
through all generations.
I will declare that your love stands firm forever,
that you have established your faithfulness in heaven itself.

Psalm 89:1–2 niv

# I am Pardoned

Where is another God like you, who pardons the sins
of the survivors among his people? You cannot
stay angry with your people, for you love to be merciful.
Once again you will have compassion on us. You will tread
our sins beneath your feet; you will throw them into
the depths of the ocean! You will bless us as you
promised Jacob long ago. You will set your love upon us,
as you promised our father Abraham!

MICAH 7:18–20 TLB

Sin shall no longer be your master,
because you are not under the law, but under grace.

ROMANS 6:14 NIV

He gives more grace. Therefore He says:

"God resists the proud,

But gives grace to the humble."

James 4:6 nkjv

God is so rich in mercy, and he loved us so much,

that even though we were dead because of our sins,

he gave us life when he raised Christ from the dead.

(It is only by God's grace that you have been saved!)…

God saved you by his grace when you believed.

And you can't take credit for this; it is a gift from God.

Salvation is not a reward for the good things we have

done, so none of us can boast about it.

Ephesians 2:4–5, 8–9 nlt

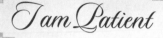

# I am Patient

The LORD longs to be gracious to you;

therefore he will rise up to show you compassion.

For the LORD is a God of justice.

Blessed are all who wait for him!

ISAIAH 30:18 NIV


The Lord isn't really being slow about his promise,

as some people think. No, he is being patient

for your sake. He does not want anyone to be destroyed,

but wants everyone to repent.

2 PETER 3:9 NLT

As a prisoner for the Lord, then, I urge you to
live a life worthy of the calling you have received.
Be completely humble and gentle; be patient,
bearing with one another in love.

EPHESIANS 4:1-2 NIV

They are those who, hearing the word, hold it fast in an
honest and good heart, and bear fruit with patience.

LUKE 8:15 ESV

We are saved by trusting. And trusting means looking
forward to getting something we don't yet have—
for a man who already has something doesn't need
to hope and trust that he will get it. But if we must keep
trusting God for something that hasn't happened yet,
it teaches us to wait patiently and confidently.

ROMANS 8:24-25 TLB

Imitate those who through faith and patience
inherit what has been promised.

HEBREWS 6:12 NIV

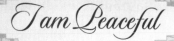

# I am Peaceful

These things I have spoken to you, so that in Me you
may have peace. In the world you have tribulation,
but take courage; I have overcome the world.

JOHN 16:33 NASB

The LORD will give strength to His people;
The LORD will bless His people with peace.

PSALM 29:11 NKJV

Peace I leave with you; my peace I give you.
I do not give to you as the world gives.
Do not let your hearts be troubled and do not be afraid.

JOHN 14:27 NIV

If people's thinking is controlled by the sinful self, there is death. But if their thinking is controlled by the Spirit, there is life and peace.

ROMANS 8:6 NCV

Those who love your instructions have great peace and do not stumble.

PSALM 119:165 NLT

God is not a God of confusion but of peace.

1 CORINTHIANS 14:33 NASB

Let the peace of Christ rule in your hearts, since as members of one body you were called to peace.

COLOSSIANS 3:15 NIV

May the Lord of peace himself give you peace at all times and in every way. The Lord be with all of you.

2 THESSALONIANS 3:16 NIV

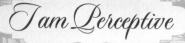
*I am Perceptive*

The unfolding of your words gives light;
it gives understanding to the simple.

PSALM 119:130 NIV

What we have received is not the spirit of the world,
but the Spirit who is from God, so that we may understand
what God has freely given us.

1 CORINTHIANS 2:12 NIV

Do not be unwise, but understand what
the will of the Lord is.

EPHESIANS 5:17 NKJV

Do not let wisdom and understanding out of your sight,
preserve sound judgment and discretion;
they will be life for you.

PROVERBS 3:21-22 NIV

Be filled with the knowledge of His will in all spiritual
wisdom and understanding, so that you will walk in
a manner worthy of the Lord… and increasing in the
knowledge of God.

Colossians 1:9-10 nasb

The wisdom from above is first of all pure.
It is also peace loving, gentle at all times, and willing
to yield to others. It is full of mercy and good deeds.
It shows no favoritism and is always sincere.

James 3:17 nlt

Listen carefully to wisdom;
set your mind on understanding.
Cry out for wisdom,
and beg for understanding.
Search for it like silver,
and hunt for it like hidden treasure.
Then you will understand respect for the Lord,
and you will find that you know God.

Proverbs 2:2-5 ncv

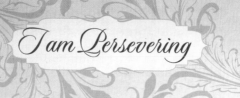

## I am Persevering

God blesses those who patiently endure testing and temptation. Afterward they will receive the crown of life that God has promised to those who love him.

JAMES 1:12 NLT

Let us not grow weary of doing good, for in due season we will reap, if we do not give up.

GALATIANS 6:9 ESV

Wait on the LORD;
Be of good courage,
And He shall strengthen your heart;
Wait, I say, on the LORD!

PSALM 27:14 NKJV

The one who endures to the end will be saved.

MATTHEW 24:13 ESV

Consider it pure joy...whenever you face trials
of many kinds, because you know that the testing
of your faith develops perseverance. Let perseverance
finish its work so that you may be mature
and complete, not lacking anything.

JAMES 1:2–4 NIV

Since we are surrounded by such a great cloud of
witnesses, let us throw off everything that hinders and
the sin that so easily entangles. And let us run with
perseverance the race marked out for us, fixing our eyes on
Jesus....so that you will not grow weary and lose heart.

HEBREWS 12:1–3 NIV

May the Lord direct your hearts into God's love
and Christ's perseverance.

2 THESSALONIANS 3:5 NIV

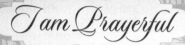

# I am Prayerful

My voice You shall hear in the morning, O LORD;

In the morning I will direct it to You,

And I will look up.

PSALM 5:3 NKJV

Ask and it will be given to you; seek and you will find;

knock and the door will be opened to you. For everyone

who asks receives; he who seeks finds; and to him who

knocks, the door will be opened.

MATTHEW 7:7–8 NIV

I call on you, My God, for you will answer me;

turn your ear to me and hear my prayer.

PSALM 17:6 NIV

The prayer of a righteous person is powerful and effective.

JAMES 5:16 NIV

The Spirit also helps our weakness; for we do not
know how to pray as we should, but the Spirit Himself
intercedes for us with groanings too deep for words.

ROMANS 8:26 NASB

Pray without ceasing.

1 THESSALONIANS 5:17 NKJV

You, God, are my God,
earnestly I seek you;
I thirst for you,
my whole being longs for you,
in a dry and parched land
where there is no water.

PSALM 63:1 NIV

With all prayer and petition pray at all times in the Spirit,
and with this in view, be on the alert with
all perseverance and petition for all the saints.

EPHESIANS 6:18 NASB

# I am Protected

The Lord himself goes before you and will be with you;

he will never leave you nor forsake you.

Deuteronomy 31:8 niv

If you make the Lord your refuge,

if you make the Most High your shelter,

no evil will conquer you;

no plague will come near your home.

For he will order his angels

to protect you wherever you go.

Psalm 91:9–11 nlt

How great is the goodness

you have stored up for those who fear you.

You lavish it on those who come to you for protection,

blessing them before the watching world.

Psalm 31:19 nlt

The Lord is faithful, and he will
strengthen you and protect you.

2 Thessalonians 3:3 niv


The Lord will keep you from all harm—
he will watch over your life;
the Lord will watch over your coming and going
both now and forevermore.

Psalm 121:7–8 niv


But let all who take refuge in you be glad;
let them ever sing for joy.
Spread your protection over them,
that those who love your name may rejoice in you.

Psalm 5:11 niv


But you, Lord, do not be far from me.
You are my strength; come quickly to help me.

Psalm 22:19 niv

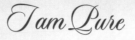
*I am Pure*

Our faces, then, are not covered. We all show the Lord's
glory, and we are being changed to be like him.
This change in us brings ever greater glory,
which comes from the Lord, who is the Spirit.

2 CORINTHIANS 3:18 NCV

Teach me your ways, O LORD,
that I may live according to your truth!
Grant me purity of heart,
so that I may honor you.

PSALM 86:11 NLT

Now that you have purified yourselves by obeying
the truth so that you have sincere love for each other,
love one another deeply, from the heart.

1 PETER 1:22 NIV

Examine everything carefully; hold fast to that which is
good; abstain from every form of evil.

1 Thessalonians 5:21-22 nasb

Whatever is true, whatever is honorable, whatever
is just, whatever is pure, whatever is lovely, whatever
is commendable, if there is any excellence, if there is
anything worthy of praise, think about these things.

Philippians 4:8 esv

Do everything without grumbling or arguing,
so that you may become blameless and pure, "children of
God without fault in a warped and crooked generation."
Then you will shine among them like stars in the sky as
you hold firmly to the word of life.

Philippians 2:14–16 niv

To do what is right and just
is more acceptable to the Lord than sacrifice.

Proverbs 21:3 niv

# I am Reconciled

You were separate from Christ...foreigners to the
covenants of the promise, without hope and without God
in the world. But now in Christ Jesus you who once were
far away have been brought near by the blood of Christ.

EPHESIANS 2:12–13 NIV

We are made right with God by placing our faith in
Jesus Christ. And this is true for everyone who believes,
no matter who we are. For everyone has sinned;
we all fall short of God's glorious standard.
Yet God, with undeserved kindness, declares that
we are righteous. He did this through Christ Jesus
when he freed us from the penalty for our sins.

ROMANS 3:22–24 NLT

We have stopped evaluating others from a human point of view. At one time we thought of Christ merely from a human point of view. How differently we know him now! This means that anyone who belongs to Christ has become a new person. The old life is gone; a new life has begun! And all of this is a gift from God, who brought us back to himself through Christ. And God has given us this task of reconciling people to him.

2 CORINTHIANS 5:16–18 NLT

# I am Redeemed

By entering through faith into what God has always
wanted to do for us—set us right with him, make us fit
for him—we have it all together with God because of
our Master Jesus. And that's not all: We throw open our
doors to God and discover at the same moment that he
has already thrown open his door to us. We find ourselves
standing where we always hoped we might stand—out in
the wide open spaces of God's grace and glory, standing
tall and shouting our praise.

ROMANS 5:1–2 MSG

Be gracious to me, O God,

according to Your lovingkindness;

According to the greatness of Your compassion

blot out my transgressions.

Psalm 51:1 nasb

Once you were dead because of your disobedience and

your many sins.... All of us used to live that way, following

the passionate desires and inclinations of our sinful

nature. By our very nature we were subject to God's anger,

just like everyone else. But God is so rich in mercy,

and he loved us so much, that even though we

were dead because of our sins, he gave us life

when he raised Christ from the dead.

Ephesians 2:1, 3–5 nlt

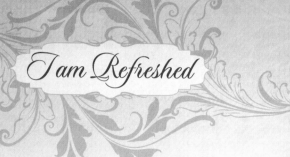

# I am Refreshed

The law of the LORD is perfect,
refreshing the soul.
The statutes of the LORD are trustworthy,
making wise the simple.

PSALM 19:7 NIV

Jesus replied that people soon became thirsty again after
drinking this water. "But the water I give them," he said,
"becomes a perpetual spring within them, watering them
forever with eternal life."

JOHN 4:13-14 TLB

A generous person will prosper;

whoever refreshes others will be refreshed.

PROVERBS 11: 25 NIV

Jesus stood and said..."Let anyone who is thirsty come to

me and drink. Whoever believes in me, as Scripture has

said, rivers of living water will flow from within them."

JOHN 7:37–38 NIV

Your love, LORD, reaches to the heavens,

your faithfulness to the skies.

Your righteousness is like the highest mountains,

your justice like the great deep.

You, LORD, preserve both people and animals.

How priceless is your unfailing love, O God!

People take refuge in the shadow of your wings.

They feast on the abundance of your house;

you give them drink from your river of delights.

For with you is the fountain of life;

in your light we see light.

PSALM 36:5–9 NIV

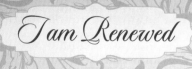

# *I am Renewed*

We shall not all sleep, but we shall all be changed.

The Lord is good to all,
and his mercy is over all that he has made.

When you were stuck in your old sin-dead life, you were
incapable of responding to God. God brought you alive—
right along with Christ! Think of it! All sins forgiven, the
slate wiped clean, that old arrest warrant canceled and
nailed to Christ's cross.

If anyone is in Christ, he is a new creation; old things have passed away; behold, all things have become new.

2 Corinthians 5:17 NKJV

Praise the Lord!
Oh, give thanks to the Lord, for He is good!
For His mercy endures forever.

Psalm 106:1 NKJV

God put the world square with himself through the Messiah, giving the world a fresh start by offering forgiveness of sins. God has given us the task of telling everyone what he is doing. We're Christ's representatives. God uses us to persuade men and women to drop their differences and enter into God's work of making things right between them. We're speaking for Christ himself now: Become friends with God; he's already a friend with you.

2 Corinthians 5:19–20 MSG

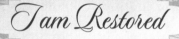
## I am Restored

Since we have been made right in God's sight by faith,
we have peace with God because of what Jesus Christ
our Lord has done for us. Because of our faith,
Christ has brought us into this place of undeserved
privilege where we now stand, and we confidently and
joyfully look forward to sharing God's glory.

ROMANS 5:1–2 NLT

He has saved us and called us to a holy life—
not because of anything we have done
but because of his own purpose and grace.

2 TIMOTHY 1:9 NIV

Dear brothers and sisters, we can boldly enter heaven's Most Holy Place because of the blood of Jesus. By his death, Jesus opened a new and life-giving way through the curtain into the Most Holy Place. And since we have a great High Priest who rules over God's house, let us go right into the presence of God with sincere hearts fully trusting him.

HEBREWS 10:19–22 NLT

Let us praise the Lord, the God of Israel, because he has come to help his people and has given them freedom.
He has given us a powerful Savior.

LUKE 1:68-69 NCV

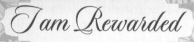

## I am Rewarded

Without faith it is impossible to please God, because
anyone who comes to him must believe that he exists and
that he rewards those who earnestly seek him.

HEBREWS 11:6 NIV

Do not lose the courage you had in the past,
which has a great reward. You must hold on, so you can
do what God wants and receive what he has promised.

HEBREWS 10:35–36 NCV

Watch yourselves, so that you may not lose what
we have worked for, but may win a full reward.

2 JOHN 1:8 ESV

Look, I am coming soon! My reward is with me, and I will

give to each person according to what they have done.

REVELATION 22:12 NIV


Remember that the Lord will reward

each one of us for the good we do.

EPHESIANS 6:8 NLT


I have fought the good fight, I have finished the course,

I have kept the faith; in the future there is laid up for me

the crown of righteousness, which the Lord, the righteous

Judge, will award to me on that day; and not only to me,

but also to all who have loved His appearing.

2 TIMOTHY 4:7-8 NASB

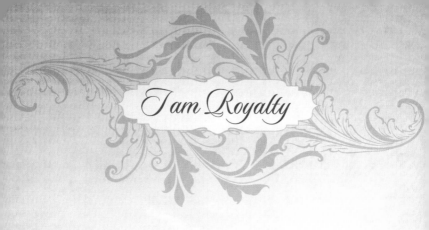

# I am Royalty

Because we are his children, God has sent the
Spirit of his Son into our hearts, prompting us
to call out, "Abba, Father." Now you are no longer
a slave but God's own child. And since you are his child,
God has made you his heir.

GALATIANS 4:6-7 NLT

As many as received Him, to them He gave
the right to become children of God,
even to those who believe in His name.

JOHN 1:12 NASB

See what great love the Father has lavished on us,

that we should be called children of God!

And that is what we are! The reason the world does not

know us is that it did not know him. Dear friends, now we

are children of God, and what we will be has not yet been

made known. But we know that when Christ appears, we

shall be like him, for we shall see him as he is.

1 JOHN 3:1-2 NIV

Love your enemies, do good to them, and lend to them

without expecting to get anything back. Then your reward

will be great, and you will be children of the Most High.

LUKE 6:35 NIV

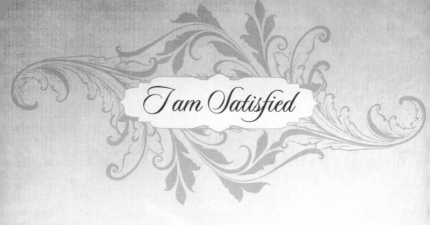

# I am Satisfied

Because your love is better than life,

my lips will glorify you.

I will praise you as long as I live,

and in your name I will lift up my hands.

I will be fully satisfied as with the richest of foods;

with singing lips my mouth will praise you.

Psalm 63:3–5 niv


God is able to provide you with every blessing in

abundance, so that by always having enough of everything,

you may share abundantly in every good work.

2 Corinthians 9:8 nrsv

The LORD is all I need.

He takes care of me.

My share in life has been pleasant;

my part has been beautiful.

PSALM 16:5–6 NCV

The poor shall eat and be satisfied; all who see

the Lord shall find him and shall praise his name.

Their hearts shall rejoice with everlasting joy.

PSALM 22:26 TLB

Give, and it will be given to you.

A good measure, pressed down, shaken together

and running over, will be poured into your lap.

For with the measure you use,

it will be measured to you.

LUKE 6:38 NIV

Whoever pursues righteousness and love

finds life, prosperity and honor.

PROVERBS 21:21 NIV

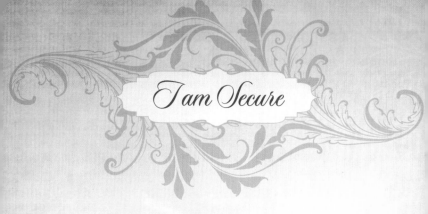

# I am Secure

The everlasting God is your place of safety,

and his arms will hold you up forever.

DEUTERONOMY 33:27 NCV

Every good and perfect gift is from above,

coming down from the Father of the heavenly lights,

who does not change like shifting shadows.

JAMES 1:17 NIV

You are near, LORD,

and all your commands are true.

Long ago I learned from your statutes

that you established them to last forever.

PSALM 119:151–152 NIV

The grass withers,

And its flower falls away,

But the word of the LORD endures forever.

1 PETER 1:24–25 NKJV


In peace I will lie down and sleep,

for you alone, LORD,

make me dwell in safety.

PSALM 4:8 NIV


When you go through deep waters and great trouble,

I will be with you. When you go through rivers

of difficulty, you will not drown! When you walk through

the fire of oppression, you will not be burned up—

the flames will not consume you.

ISAIAH 43:2 TLB


Our steps are made firm by the LORD,

when he delights in our way;

though we stumble, we shall not fall headlong,

for the LORD holds us by the hand.

PSALM 37:23–24 NRSV

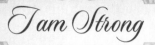

# I am Strong

Have you never heard?

Have you never understood?

The LORD is the everlasting God,

the Creator of all the earth.

He never grows weak or weary.

No one can measure the depths of his understanding.

He gives power to the weak

and strength to the powerless.

Even youths will become weak and tired,

and young men will fall in exhaustion.

But those who trust in the LORD will find new strength.

They will soar high on wings like eagles.

They will run and not grow weary.

They will walk and not faint.

ISAIAH 40:28-31 NLT

"My grace is sufficient for you, for My strength is made perfect in weakness." Therefore most gladly I will rather boast in my infirmities, that the power of Christ may rest upon me…. For when I am weak, then I am strong.

2 CORINTHIANS 12:9 NKJV

In Your hand is power and might;
In Your hand it is to make great
And to give strength to all.

1 CHRONICLES 29:12 NKJV

Be strong in the Lord and in his mighty power.
Put on the full armor of God, so that you can
take your stand against the devil's schemes.

EPHESIANS 6:10–11 NIV

# I am Supported

The Lord stood by me and gave me strength....
The Lord will rescue me from every evil attack
and save me for his heavenly kingdom.

2 TIMOTHY 4:17-18 NRSV


Whom have I in heaven but you?
And earth has nothing I desire besides you.
My flesh and my heart may fail,
but God is the strength of my heart
and my portion forever.

PSALM 73:25–26 NIV


The LORD is near to the brokenhearted
and saves the crushed in spirit.

PSALM 34:18 ESV

You, God, see the trouble of the afflicted;
you consider their grief and take it in hand.
The victims commit themselves to you;
you are the helper of the fatherless.

Psalm 10:14 niv

Live as citizens of heaven, conducting yourselves in
a manner worthy of the Good News about Christ...
standing together with one spirit and one purpose,
fighting together for the faith. Don't be intimidated in any
way by your enemies. This will be a sign to them that you
are going to be saved, even by God himself.

Philippians 1:27–28 nlt

God will never forget the needy;
the hope of the afflicted will never perish.

Psalm 9:18 niv

You are my hiding place;
You shall preserve me from trouble;
You shall surround me with songs of deliverance.

Psalm 32:7 nkjv

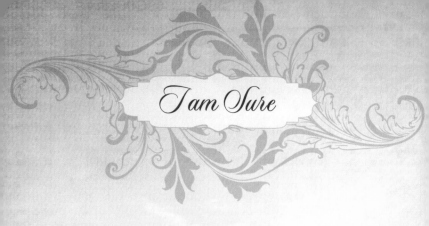

## I am Sure

Faith is confidence in what we hope for
and assurance about what we do not see.

HEBREWS 11:1 NIV

Not one word of all the good words which the LORD
your God spoke concerning you has failed; all have been
fulfilled for you, not one of them has failed.

JOSHUA 23:14 NASB

As we pray to our God and Father about you, we think of
your faithful work, your loving deeds, and the enduring
hope you have because of our Lord Jesus Christ.

1 THESSALONIANS 1:3 NLT

Faith comes by hearing, and hearing by the word of God.

ROMANS 10:17 NKJV

If you have faith like a grain of mustard seed, you will say to this mountain, "Move from here to there," and it will move, and nothing will be impossible for you.

MATTHEW 17:20 ESV

Through Christ you have come to trust in God. And you have placed your faith and hope in God because he raised Christ from the dead and gave him great glory.

1 PETER 1:21 NLT

Until heaven and earth disappear, not the smallest letter, not the least stroke of a pen, will by any means disappear from the Law until everything is accomplished.

MATTHEW 5:18 NIV

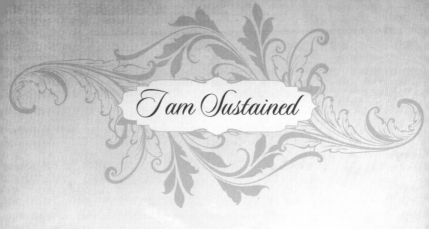

# I am Sustained

God is able to bless you abundantly, so that
in all things at all times, having all that you need,
you will abound in every good work.

2 Corinthians 9:8 NIV

The Lord is my shepherd, I shall not want.
He makes me lie down in green pastures;
he leads me beside still waters;
he restores my soul.

Psalm 23:1–3 NRSV

You're blessed when you're at the end of your rope.
With less of you there is more of God and his rule.

Matthew 5:3 msg

I fall to my knees and pray to the Father, the Creator of
everything in heaven and on earth.
I pray that from his glorious, unlimited resources he will
empower you with inner strength through his Spirit. Then
Christ will make his home in your hearts as you trust in
him. Your roots will grow down into God's love and keep
you strong. And may you have the power to understand,
as all God's people should, how wide, how long, how high,
and how deep his love is. May you experience the love of
Christ, though it is too great to understand fully. Then
you will be made complete with all the fullness of life and
power that comes from God.

Ephesians 3:14–19 nlt

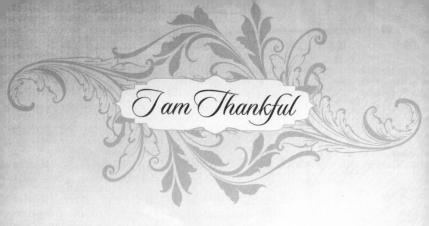

# I am Thankful

That my soul may sing praise to You and not be silent.
O LORD my God, I will give thanks to You forever.

PSALM 30:12 NASB

Thanks be to God for his indescribable gift!

2 CORINTHIANS 9:15 NIV

Be filled with the Holy Spirit, singing psalms and hymns
and spiritual songs among yourselves, and making music
to the Lord in your hearts. And give thanks for everything
to God the Father in the name of our Lord Jesus Christ.

EPHESIANS 5:18–20 NLT

Give thanks to the LORD, for he is good.

His love endures forever.

PSALM 136:1 NIV


Always be thankful. Let the message about Christ, in all
its richness, fill your lives. Teach and counsel each other
with all the wisdom he gives. Sing psalms and hymns and
spiritual songs to God with thankful hearts. And whatever
you do or say, do it as a representative of the Lord Jesus,
giving thanks through him to God the Father.

COLOSSIANS 3:15-17 NLT


In everything give thanks; for this is God's will
for you in Christ Jesus.

1 THESSALONIANS 5:18 NASB


Now therefore, our God,
We thank You
And praise Your glorious name.

1 CHRONICLES 29:13 NKJV

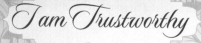

# I am Trustworthy

Listen, for I will speak of excellent things,
And from the opening of my lips will come right things;
For my mouth will speak truth.

PROVERBS 8:6–7 NKJV

One who is faithful in a very little is also faithful in much.

LUKE 16:10 ESV

You must remain faithful to the things you have been taught.
You know they are true, for you know you can trust those
who taught you. You have been taught the holy Scriptures
from childhood, and they have given you the wisdom to
receive the salvation that comes by trusting in Christ Jesus.

2 TIMOTHY 3:14–15 NLT

The LORD detests lying lips,
but he delights in people who are trustworthy.

PROVERBS 12:22 NIV

A gossip goes around telling secrets,
but those who are trustworthy can keep a confidence.

PROVERBS 11:13 NLT

Show yourself in all respects to be a model of good works,
and in your teaching show integrity, dignity, and sound
speech that cannot be condemned, so that an opponent
may be put to shame, having nothing evil to say about us.

TITUS 2:7-8 ESV

Love and truth form a good leader;
sound leadership is founded on loving integrity.

PROVERBS 20:28 MSG

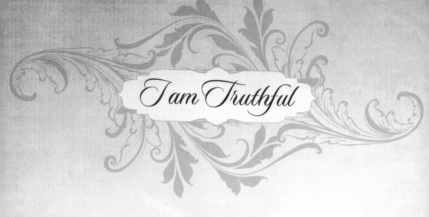

# I am Truthful

Truthful words stand the test of time,

but lies are soon exposed.

PROVERBS 12:19 NLT

When he, the Spirit of truth, comes,

he will guide you into all the truth.

JOHN 16:13 NIV

You desire truth in the innermost being,

And in the hidden part You will make me know wisdom.

PSALM 51:6 NASB

Let us not love with words or speech

but with actions and in truth.

1 JOHN 3:18 NIV

The very essence of your words is truth;
all your just regulations will stand forever.

PSALM 119:160 NLT

Everyone who does evil hates the light, and will not come
into the light for fear that their deeds will be exposed.
But whoever lives by the truth comes into the light,
so that it may be seen plainly that what they have
done has been done in the sight of God.

JOHN 3:20–21 NIV

His merciful kindness is great toward us,
And the truth of the LORD endures forever.
Praise the LORD!

PSALM 117:2 NKJV

Send out your light and your truth;
let them lead me;
let them bring me to your holy hill
and to your dwelling.

PSALM 43:3 NRSV

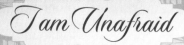
## I am Unafraid

There is no room in love for fear. Well-formed love banishes fear. Since fear is crippling, a fearful life—fear of death, fear of judgment—is one not yet fully formed in love.

1 JOHN 4:18 MSG

Don't be afraid, for I am with you.
Don't be discouraged, for I am your God.
I will strengthen you and help you.
I will hold you up with my victorious right hand.

ISAIAH 41:10 NLT

God has not given us a spirit of fear,
but of power and of love and of a sound mind.

2 TIMOTHY 1:7 NKJV

The LORD is my light and my salvation;
whom shall I fear?
The LORD is the stronghold of my life;
of whom shall I be afraid?

PSALM 27:1 ESV

Say to those with fearful hearts,
"Be strong, and do not fear,
for your God...is coming to save you."

ISAIAH 35:4 NLT

When you lie down, you will not be afraid;
when you lie down, your sleep will be sweet.
Have no fear of sudden disaster
or of the ruin that overtakes the wicked,
for the LORD will be at your side
and will keep your foot from being snared.

PROVERBS 3:24–26 NIV

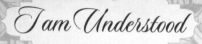

## I am Understood

You know what I long for, Lord;

you hear my every sigh.

PSALM 38:9 NLT

My sheep hear my voice, and I know them, and they

follow me. I give them eternal life, and they will never

perish, and no one will snatch them out of my hand.

JOHN 10:27-28 ESV

God is not unjust; he will not overlook your work and the

love that you showed for his sake in

serving the saints, as you still do.

HEBREWS 6:10 NRSV

Your Father knows what you need before you ask Him.

MATTHEW 6:8 NASB

Great is our Lord and mighty in power;
his understanding has no limit.

PSALM 147:5 NIV


For we do not have a high priest who is unable to empathize
with our weaknesses, but we have one who has been
tempted in every way, just as we are—yet he did not sin.

HEBREWS 4:15 NIV


As the heavens are higher than the earth,
So are My ways higher than your ways
And My thoughts higher than your thoughts.

ISAIAH 55:9 NASB


Blessed is the one who finds wisdom,
and the one who gets understanding.

PROVERBS 3:13 ESV


Our purpose is to please God, not people. He alone
examines the motives of our hearts.

1 THESSALONIANS 2:4 NLT

# I am Untroubled

Blessed is the one who trusts in the LORD,

whose confidence is in him.

They will be like a tree planted by the water

that sends out its roots by the stream.

It does not fear when heat comes;

its leaves are always green.

It has no worries in a year of drought

and never fails to bear fruit.

JEREMIAH 17:7–8 NIV

Let not your heart be troubled; you believe in God, believe also in Me. In My Father's house are many mansions.... I go to prepare a place for you. And if I go and prepare a place for you, I will come again and receive you to Myself; that where I am, there you may be also.

John 14:1-3 nkjv

Give your entire attention to what God is doing right now, and don't get worked up about what may or may not happen tomorrow. God will help you deal with whatever hard things come up when the time comes.

Matthew 6:34 msg

Those who love me, I will deliver;
I will protect those who know my name.
When they call to me, I will answer them;
I will be with them in trouble,
I will rescue them and honor them.

Psalm 91:14-15 nrsv

# I am Unwavering

Be attentive to my words;

incline your ear to my sayings.

Let them not escape from your sight;

keep them within your heart.

Let your eyes look directly forward,

and your gaze be straight before you.

Proverbs 4:20–21, 25 esv

Let us draw near to God with a sincere heart and with the

full assurance that faith brings….Let us hold unswervingly

to the hope we profess, for he who promised is faithful.

Hebrews 10:22-23 niv

Your lovingkindness, O Lord, extends to the heavens,

Your faithfulness reaches to the skies.

Psalm 36:5 nasb

God is faithful. He will not allow the temptation to be
more than you can stand. When you are tempted,
he will show you a way out so that you can endure.

1 Corinthians 10:13 nlt

I keep my eyes always on the Lord.
With him at my right hand, I will not be shaken.

Psalm 16:8 niv

Lord, you are my God;
I will exalt you and praise your name,
for in perfect faithfulness
you have done wonderful things,
things planned long ago.

Isaiah 25:1 niv

The word of the Lord is upright,
and all his work is done in faithfulness.

Psalm 33:4 esv

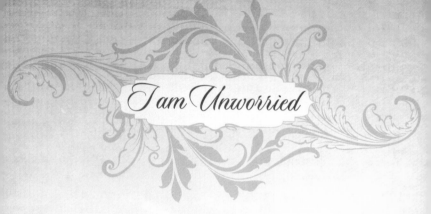

# I am Unworried

Which of you by worrying can add
a single hour to his life's span?

LUKE 12:25 NASB

Don't worry about anything; instead, pray about
everything. Tell God what you need, and thank him for all
he has done. Then you will experience God's peace, which
exceeds anything we can understand. His peace will guard
your hearts and minds as you live in Christ Jesus.

PHILIPPIANS 4:6–7 NLT

Worry weighs a person down;
an encouraging word cheers a person up.

PROVERBS 12:25 NLT

Give your burdens to the LORD,
and he will take care of you.

PSALM 55:22 NLT

Do not worry about your life, what you will eat or drink;
or about your body, what you will wear. Is not life more
than food, and the body more than clothes? Look at the
birds of the air; they do not sow or reap or store away in
barns, and yet your heavenly Father feeds them. Are you
not much more valuable than they?

MATTHEW 6:25–26 NIV

May the Lord of peace himself give you peace at all times
in every way.

2 THESSALONIANS 3:16 ESV

If people's thinking is controlled by the sinful self, there
is death. But if their thinking is controlled by the Spirit,
there is life and peace.

ROMANS 8:6 NCV

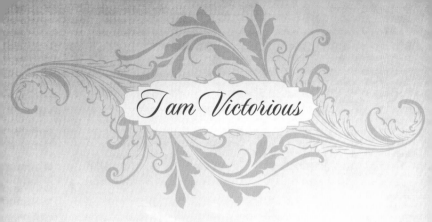

## I am Victorious

Thanks be to God! He gives us the victory
through our Lord Jesus Christ.

1 Corinthians 15:57 niv

Can anything ever separate us from Christ's love?
Does it mean he no longer loves us if we have trouble
or calamity, or are persecuted, or hungry, or destitute,
or in danger, or threatened with death?
No, despite all these things, overwhelming victory is
ours through Christ, who loved us.

Romans 8:35, 37 nlt

Commit your actions to the Lord,
and your plans will succeed.

Proverbs 16:3 nlt

Thanks be to God, who always leads us in triumph
in Christ, and manifests through us the sweet aroma
of the knowledge of Him in every place.

2 Corinthians 2:14 nasb

In fact, this is love for God: to keep his commands.
And his commands are not burdensome, for everyone
born of God overcomes the world. This is the victory
that has overcome the world, even our faith. Who is it that
overcomes the world? Only the one who believes
that Jesus is the Son of God.

1 John 5:3-5 niv

Victory comes from you, O Lord.
May you bless your people.

Psalm 3:8 nlt

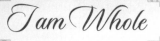

# I am Whole

God made my life complete
when I placed all the pieces before him....
God rewrote the text of my life
when I opened the book of my heart to his eyes.

Psalm 18:20, 24 msg

For you who fear my name, the sun of righteousness shall
rise with healing in its wings.

Malachi 4:2 esv

He will take our weak mortal bodies and change them
into glorious bodies like his own, using the same power
with which he will bring everything under his control.

Philippians 3:21 nlt

What a God we have! And how fortunate we are to have him, this Father of our Master Jesus! Because Jesus was raised from the dead, we've been given a brand-new life and have everything to live for, including a future in heaven—and the future starts now! God is keeping careful watch over us and the future. The Day is coming when you'll have it all—life healed and whole.

1 Peter 1:3–5 msg

This is how much God loved the world:
He gave his Son, his one and only Son.
And this is why: so that no one need be destroyed;
by believing in him, anyone can have
a whole and lasting life.

John 3:16 msg